PIRATE AND BUCCANEER DOCTORS

Leo Eloesser

COACHWHIP PUBLICATIONS

Greenville, Ohio

Pirate and Buccaneer Doctors, by Leo Eloesser
Leo Eloesser (1881-1976)

© 2013 Coachwhip Publications
No claim made on public domain material.

Cover: Pirate symbol © Stanislav Paramonov; Medical symbol
    © Prokhor Korolkov

ISBN 1-61646-186-1
ISBN-13 978-1-61646-186-7

CoachwhipBooks.com

PIRATE AND BUCCANEER DOCTORS
Leo Eloesser
Annals of Medical History
Vol. 8, No. 1, March 1926, pp. 31-60

PIRATE AND BUCCANEER DOCTORS

By LEO ELOESSER, M.D.

SAN FRANCISCO, CALIFORNIA

IF romance lie in encounters with the unknown, whether that unknown be in the depths of a man's own heart, as in the romance of love, or in foreign circumstance, as in the romance of battle and adventure, then the present quickening of interest in sailing ships and older matters of the sea is understandable and praiseworthy.

For yearnings toward romance will never die in the spirits of boys and men who, if they cannot find romance in the present, will seek it in the past.

And sailing ships are among the last of the natural encounterers of the unknown; their masts and yards, lacing the skyline of the former San Francisco waterfront, lie unforgotten within the memories of even the younger of us.

There is little of the unknown left to encounter: Rockwell Kent had to go to the ends of the earth, to Tierra del Fuego, to find it. Science, perfection of mechanics and mathematical calculation are driving adventure to the wall. There are no longer uncharted seas. The very air currents will soon be charted, and adventure be a matter of capacity of gas-tanks and strength of fuselage. When Andrews was asked what adventures had befallen him in the Gobi desert, he replied that he had had no adventures, that adventures were a confession of poor calculation or unpreparedness.

Yes, Romance of Adventure will disappear, if it has not already done so; it will find a puny substitute in Romance of the Soul, in men's boring about in the objects and subjects of their own emotions and desires; an onanistic tickling of their own and their neighbor's navels; or in more or less melancholy reflections over deeds and adventures of the past.

So we who have looked down from Telegraph Hill and have seen a gently swaying forest of masts girdle old wooden docks, and have stood on the cliffs at Baker's Beach and watched square-rigged ships, all sails set, bear down past hovering pilot boats into the Golden Gate, think longingly of these last adventurers and of the brave lives that disappeared with them.

A certain romantic inclination of my own and a confidence in the same bent in others, then, are my reasons for discovering to the readers of the ANNALS OF MEDICAL HISTORY the names, at least, of some of their hardier old colleagues.

Every one knows what a Pirate is. The line dividing him from a Buccaneer is a hazy one, yet there is a faint and hazy line. A pirate scrupled not whom he would make his prize; the buccaneers were originally French and English cattle hunters settled on the Island of Tortuga near Haiti, whose hereditary enemy and prey were the Spanish. Later they enlisted with them Dutch and occasionally Portuguese. Their warfare was at first legitimate; during the war between England and Spain they sailed under English or Jamaican letters of marque. The intricacies of the various outbreaks of war, treaties of peace and armistices, their application north and east of the line and their ineffectiveness south and west of it are too complex to be related here. Let it suffice that from about 1630, when we first begin to hear of buccaneers, until 1697, when the last legally countenanced privateering expedition under Sieur de Pointis set sail from France and took Cartagena with a force composed of Frenchmen and of Haitian buccaneers, most buccaneers made some effort to equip themselves with papers that would lend to their raids a show of legitimate warfare. It is true that many of the papers ill stood scrutiny. Some were little better than fishing licenses. Here is what Esquemeling relates of the commission under which the first great buccaneering fleet ravaged the Pacific and laid siege to Panama.

We shewed him our commission, which was now for three years to come. This we had purchased at a cheap rate, having given for it only the sum of ten ducats, or pieces-of-eight. But the truth of the thing was that at first our commission was made only for the space of three months, the same date as the Frenchman's was; whereas among ourselves we had contrived to make it last for three years—for with this we were resolved to seek our fortunes.[1]

In 1670 a treaty of peace was concluded between England and Spain, and more or less hearty attempts were made by Jamaican governors to enforce it in the West Indies and on the Spanish Main. After this English vessels pretending to legitimacy were forced to seek papers from the French colony in Hispaniola or from some of the smaller English West Indies where piratical governors still issued privateering letters in defiance of orders from the main colony.

The way of the buccaneers grew harder and harder; those of them who chose to continue their depredations upon their hereditary Spanish enemy sailed without papers. Some sought refuge in the North American colonies; the governor of North Carolina in particular seemed disposed to shut a friendly eye to piracy and to profit by booty brought into Carolinian ports and rivers. Other raiders made their way across the Isthmus of Panama to the South Seas where they harassed the west coasts of South and Central America without fear of surveillance.

The heyday of buccaneering lay in the last half of the seventeenth century. The eyes of the buccaneer were first opened to the riches of the sea by Pierre le Grand who, some time between 1630 and 1640, boarded a Spanish galleon from a small boat:

The boat, . . . wherein Pierre le Grand was with his companions, had now been at sea a long time, without finding anything according to his intent of piracy suitable to make a prey. And now, their provisions beginning to fail, they could keep themselves no longer upon the ocean or they must of necessity starve. Being almost

[1] Esquemeling. The Buccaneers of America. Lond. and N. Y., p. 257-258.

reduced to despair, they espied a great ship belonging to the Spanish flota which had separated from the rest. This bulky vessel they resolved to set upon and take, or die in the attempt. Hereupon they made sail towards her, with design to view her strength. And, although they judged the vessel to be far above their forces, yet the covetousness of such a prey and the extremity of fortune they were reduced unto, made them adventure upon such an enterprise. Being now come so near that they could not escape without danger of being all killed, the Pirates jointly made an oath unto their captain, Pierre le Grand, to behave themselves courageously in this attempt without the least fear or fainting. True it is that these rovers had conceived an opinion they should find the ship unprovided to fight, and that through this occasion they should master her by degrees. It was in the dusk of the evening, or soon after, when this great action was performed. But, before it was begun, they gave orders unto the surgeon of the boat to bore a hole in the sides thereof, to the intent that, their own vessel sinking under them, they might be compelled to attack more vigorously and endeavour more hastily to run aboard the great ship. This was performed accordingly; and without any other arms than a pistol in one of their hands and a sword in the other, they immediately climbed up the sides of the ship, and ran altogether into the great cabin, where they found the Captain, with several of his companions, playing at cards. Here they set a pistol to his breast, commanding him to deliver up the ship unto their obedience. The Spaniards, seeing the Pirates aboard their ship, without scarce having seen them at sea, cried out: "Jesus bless us! Are these devils or what are they?" In the meanwhile, some of them took possession of the gun-room, and seized the arms and military affairs they found there, killing as many of the ship as made opposition. By which means the Spaniards presently were compelled to surrender. . . .

The planters and hunters of the isle of Tortuga had no sooner understood this happy event, and the rich prize those pirates had obtained, but they resolved to follow their example.[2]

Piracy, directed mainly against the Spaniards, continued to flourish for another thirty

[2] Esquemeling. *Op. cit.*, pp. 56-57.

years. Woodes-Rogers, appointed Governor of the Bahamas in 1718, managed to stamp it out in the West Indies by dint of a combination of pardons, clemency and hangings. He must have been a rare sea captain to have kept the respect and love of his unruly subjects while carrying out his hard task.

For the pirate of that day occupied much the place of the rum-runner in this. The law dealt hard with him, but the citizenry were all on his side; he flung his gains about him in Jamaican ports with a profligate hand; merchants, inn-keepers and ladies of the town took his disbursements kindly; officials filled their coffers with his tithes, connived at his escape and hanged him, when they had to, with regret. And as for the pirate himself, he regarded forays upon Spanish towns and the capture of Spanish ships as legitimate enterprise. Why should a scrap of paper turn his hereditary enemy into a *noli me tangere* and outlaw a profession which both governors and governments had used in time of need? A Spaniard was a Spaniard, treaty or none.

Treaties, peace and governors turned respectable buccaneers and privateers into wholly unrespectable pirates. So it is with the habit of man-hunting; once acquired it seems hard to break: the aftermath of 1914–1918 is not so very different.

Wherefore, in spite of Woodes-Rogers, hangings, laws and pursuits, pirates continued to flourish well into the eighteenth century. And seeing that they were to be hanged anyway, they grew less nice about the nationality of their prizes. Every ship was their foe and they were every ship's; they spread from the West Indies and ravaged the Indian Ocean and the African slave coasts. On Madagascar they established settlements and made various ocean islands their strongholds. Captain Avery, who took the Great Mogul's own ship and in her an Indian princess, whose name in the year 1715–1716 was in every man's mouth, a sort of eighteenth century yellow journal hero; Capt. Bartholomew Roberts, who commanded pirate ships from February, 1720, until February 10, 1722, when in a battle with the man-of-war Swallow, "Death, who took a swift passage in a grape shot . . . struck him directly on the throat"; Captain Edward Teach (Blackbeard), one of the most ferocious of pirates, 1717–1718, pet of the Carolinian governor, whom Lieutenant Maynard engaged in fierce hand-to-hand combat in Ockerekoke Inlet, North Carolina, bearing back, hanging from the bowsprit of his sloop, the slain pirate's head; William Kidd, who scarcely merits his renown, a vacillating character who, though he doubtless deserved the hanging that he got, was hanged as a sop to politics; these were the most famous.

It was not law or governments that killed piracy, but steam. Piracy lasted until the beginning of the last century; one of its finest and most generously romantic figures was Jean Lafitte, the Louisianian pirate. During the War of 1812, he was approached by the English; but he scorned their overtures and offered his services to the United States, fighting with his men by the side of General Jackson at the battle of New Orleans. In 1815 he was pardoned by President Monroe in consideration of his services during this battle. Later he made his headquarters in Galveston and, falling again into piracy, was said to have been killed in a fight with a British sloop of war.

Thus we have tried rapidly to sketch the rise and fall of buccaneering and piracy.

The buccaneers were a romantic crew. They took their name from the *boucan*, i.e., jerking meat over a slow smudge, a process they had from the native Caribbees. They lived originally by hunting wild cattle, for which purpose they would disappear from their settlements into the forests of Northern Haiti for a year or more at a time. They were clad in blouses and drawers, black and stiff with the gore of slaughtered cattle. These bloody vestments they never changed but wore as a proud uniform. The achievement of Pierre le Grand suddenly opened their eyes to the fortunes that were sailing away from under their grasp; they saw that cattle rustling was but a slow way of getting rich; and after Pierre's exploit there was a mad rush from the Island of Tortuga into any kind of a vessel that would bear men against the Spaniard. A veritable Klondike rush.

Both buccaneers and pirates were joined in a democratic community, sailing under a code known as the "Jamaica Discipline." They had furthermore a set of articles varying a little under different commanders and in different expeditions.

Captain Bartholomew Roberts' articles read as follows:

Captain Bartholomew Roberts' Articles

I

Every man has a vote in affairs of moment, has equal title to the fresh provisions or strong liquors at any time seized, and may use them at pleasure, unless a scarcity [no uncommon thing among them] make it necessary for the good of all to vote a retrenchment.

II

Every man to be called fairly in turn by list, on board of prizes, because, over and above their proper share, they were on these occasions allowed a shift of clothes. But if they defrauded the company to the value of a dollar, in plate, jewels, or money, marooning was their punishment. [This was a barbarous custom of putting the offender on shore, on some desolate or uninhabited cape or island, with a gun, a few shot, a bottle of water, a bottle of powder, to subsist with or starve.] If the robbery was only between one another, they contented themselves with slitting the ears and nose of him that was guilty, and set him on shore, not in an uninhabited place, but somewhere where he was sure to encounter hardships.

III

No person to game at cards or dice for money.

IV

The lights and candles to be put out at eight o'clock at night. If any of the crew after that hour still remained inclined for drinking, they were to do it on the open deck. [Which Roberts believed would give a check to their debauches, for he was a sober man himself, but found at length that all his endeavours to put an end to this debauch proved ineffectual.]

V

To keep their piece, pistols and cutlass clean, and fit for service. [In this they were extravagantly nice, endeavouring to outdo one another in the beauty and richness of their arms, giving sometimes at auction at the mast £30 or £40 a pair for pistols. These were slung in time of service, with different coloured ribbons, over the shoulders, in a way peculiar to these fellows, in which they took great delight.]

VI

No boy or woman to be allowed amongst them. If any man were found seducing any of the latter sex, and carried her to sea disguised, he was to suffer death. [So that when any fell into their hands, as it chanced in the Onslow, they put a sentinel immediately over her to prevent ill consequences from so dangerous an instrument of division and quarrel; but then here lies the roguery, they contend who shall be sentinel, which happens generally to one of the greatest bullies, who, to secure the lady's virtue, will let none lie with her but himself.]

VII

To desert the ship or their quarters in battle was punished with death, or marooning.

VIII

No striking one another on board, but every man's quarrels to be ended on shore, at sword and pistol. Thus the quartermaster of the ship, when the parties will not come to any reconciliation, accompanies them on shore with what assistance he thinks proper, and turns the disputants back to back at so many paces distance. At the word of command they turn and fire immediately, or else the piece is knocked out of their hands. If both miss, they come to their cutlasses, and then he is declared victor who draws the first blood.

IX

No man to talk of breaking up their way of living till each had shared £1000. If, in order to do this, any man should lose a limb, or become a cripple in their service, he was to have 800 dollars out of the public stock, and for lesser hurts proportionably.

X

The captain and quartermaster to receive two shares of a prize; the master, boatswain, and gunner, one share and a half, and other officers one and a quarter.

XI

The musicians to have rest on the Sabbath-Day, but the other six days and nights none without special favour.[3]

Captain Ed Low's articles, and also Captain George Lowther's, read:

CAPTAIN LOWTHER'S ARTICLES

I

The Captain is to have two full Shares; the Master is to have one Share and a half; the Doctor, Mate, Gunner, and Boatswain, one Share and a quarter.

II

He that shall be found guilty of taking up any unlawful Weapon on Board the Privateer, or any prize, by us taken, so as to strike or abuse one another, in any regard, shall suffer what Punishment the Captain and Majority of the Company shall think fit.

III

He that shall be found Guilty of Cowardice, in the Time of Engagement, shall suffer what Punishment the Captain and Majority shall think fit.

IV

If any Gold, Jewels, Silver, &c. be found on Board any Prize or Prizes, to the Value of a Piece of Eight, and the Finder do not deliver it to the Quarter-Master, in the Space of 24 Hours, shall suffer what Punishment the Captain and the Majority of the Company shall think fit.

V

He that is found Guilty of Gaming, or Defrauding another to the Value of a Shilling, shall suffer what Punishment the Captain and the Majority of the Company shall think fit.

VI

He that shall have the Misfortune to lose a limb, in Time of Engagement, shall have the Sum of one hundred and fifty Pounds Sterling, and remain with the Company as long as he shall think fit.

VII

Good Quarters to be given when call'd for.

VIII

He that sees a Sail first, shall have the best Pistol, or Small-Arm, on board her.[4]

These articles were in more ways than one the forerunners of the code of modern industrial accident commissions. The wounded and disabled were allowed compensation; and although pirates and buccaneers sailed under the law of "No prey, no pay," the wounded were recompensed out of the common stock before any other division of it was made among the rest of the crew.

They stipulate in writing what recompense or reward each one ought to have that is either wounded or maimed in his body, suffering the loss of any limb, by that voyage. Thus they order for the loss of a right arm 600 pieces-of-eight, or 6 slaves; for the loss of a left arm 500 pieces-of-eight, or 5 slaves; for a right leg 500 pieces-of-eight, or 5 slaves; for a left leg, 400 pieces-of-eight, or 4 slaves; for an eye 100 pieces-of-eight, or one slave; for a finger of the hand the same reward as for the eye."[5]

"In addition to this compensation," Masefield says, "a wounded man received a crown a day (say three shillings) for two months after division of the spoil."[6]

With the buccaneers, the surgeon seems to have had a salary: "Also [they draw out of the common stock] a competent salary for the surgeon and his chest of medicaments, which usually is rated at 200 or 250 pieces-of-eight (dollars)."[7]

[3] Capt. Chas. Johnson. Quoted in Buccaneers and Marooners of America, ed. and illus. by H. Pyle, Lond., 1897, p. 289–290.

[4] Dow and Edmunds. Pirates of the New England Coast. Salem, Mass., 1923, p. 133.

[5] Esquemeling. *Op. cit.*, p. 60.

[6] Masefield, J. On the Spanish Main. Ed. 2, Lond., 1922, p. 97.

[7] Esquemeling. *Op. cit.*, p. 60.

With the pirates, the surgeon together with the mate, gunner and boatswain drew a share and a quarter of the prize. In ships engaged in legalized privateering the chirurgeon was a regular officer.

He had to bring on board his own instruments and medicines, and to keep them ready to hand in his cabin beneath the gun-deck, out of all possible reach of shot. He was expected to know his business, and to know the remedies for those ailments peculiar to the lands for which the ship intended. He had to produce a certificate from "able men of his profession" to show that he was fit to be employed. An assistant, or servant, was allowed him, and neither he, nor his servant, did any duty outside of the chirurgeon's province (Monson).[8]

The pirate surgeon, however, does not seem to have had to sign the articles. He was taken off a prize and forced to serve until another prize was taken that had a surgeon on board; he was then given his liberty, if he chose, and the new surgeon put in his place.

Peter Scudamore, Captain Roberts' surgeon, who was hanged at Cape Coast Castle in 1722, gloried in having been the first doctor to sign pirates' articles and in being as staunch and ready a pirate as the rest. We shall have more of Doctor Peter later.

It is touching to see how these rude and bloody men hung upon their doctors; how helpless they felt when cast adrift without one. It gives one a pride in his calling to see how the most arrant rascals among the doctors were honoured, and what privileges and exemptions their doctorate secured to the worst of them. For truly in a professional light, one can see little ground for the pirates' faith and trust. It was a child's and a savage's faith in a medicine-man, in magical healing plaisters and salves. The learnedest of the doctors, the lettered and studied ones among them, seem to have been a lazy, boozing and rascally lot; it was the humbler ones, who had picked up their surgery from apprenticeships, the irregular and unli-censed practitioners, whose meagerly told lives give glimpses of humanity and kindliness and readiness to help.

Before we try to evoke the pictures of a few, of whose lives we have some detail, let me call from Hades the shadowy outlines or a fleeting glimpse, a passage or two in the careers, of some of the dimmer figures among these swashbuckler surgeons.

On the fifth of April of 1680, there landed on the Atlantic side of the Isthmus of Darien a crew of 331 men under seven captains, to wit: Coxon, Harris, Sawkins, Sharp, Cook, Alleston and Macket. The sum of their designs was "to descend by the river of Darien, or any other, into the South Sea, and there to rove up and down until such time as we could meet any rich prize, or galleon coming from Lima to Panama, or else to plunder again either the city of Panama or any other of so many rich towns and villages as are known to border upon the coasts of that sea."[9] After many adventures they reached the shores of the Pacific and embarked toward Panama in a fleet of canoes. They met several Spanish sail, which they captured, and with them blockaded Panama:

Being almost ready to raise the blockade of Panama, Captain John Coxon [or Croxon] began to vary in his resolutions, and at last openly to mutiny against the rest of the Company: the effect hereof was that he departed from us and returned back with the Emperor and his son King Golden-Cap and all the Indians and canoes they had brought with them, and carrying also with him 50 of our English company and the best surgeon of the fleet, who belonged unto him and who would not go without his instruments to work withal, that is to say the medicaments, which we very much wanted for our wounded men. What medicines he left behind were not considerable in comparison of what he carried away; but this point we knew not till afterwards, or we should have torn in pieces the said surgeon and his master rather than have parted with those things of which we had so much necessity.

[8] Masefield. *Op. cit.,* p. 254.

[9] Esquemeling. *Op. cit.,* p. 261–262.

This piece of dishonesty of Captain Coxon weakened much our forces and diminished in great measure our number; for, had he taken care of or carried away our wounded men, we should not much have resented his departure, the Indians being of no considerable help unto us. But here, that he may be known, I will not omit to tell you that the chief occasion of his grudge against us was because we reproached him for his ill-behaviour in the engagement we had with the Armadilla of Panama; for in that dangerous action, to speak it all in a word, he shewed himself more like a coward than one of our profession, that is to say a true Buccaneer.

. . . Captain Coxon, who commanded in chief, being separated or departed from us, we chose in his place Captain Sawkins and Captain Sharp to lead us, and were now reduced unto 200 men, whereof many, as was said before, lay dangerously wounded in the hospital vessel.

Having, therefore, refitted ourselves at the island of Tobago, which is situated over-against the road of Panama, we sailed thence about the middle of May, 1680, in quest of some other purchase or design, coasting the shore towards the Northern parts of America commonly called California.[10]

After eight or ten days they arrived at the island of Coiba (Quiblo) and issuing thence attempted the town of Puebla Nueva. Here Captain Sawkins, the best beloved and most valiant of their commanders, in boarding a breast works, was killed. His death gave rise to new dissensions.

About ninety of his party left and returned overland. The remainder sailed along the South American coast and after sundry adventures and dissensions landed on the Isle of Juan Fernandez, where, about Christmas of 1680, they deposed Captain Sharp and elected Captain John Watling in his stead. Watling was a hymn-singing pirate and a precious poor commander; he immediately got his party into trouble and paid for it with his life.

We landed at Arica, and fought the town with 93 men, which number was all we could conveniently spare. We got into the town and took several of their breast-works, yet were repulsed

from the castle, and afterwards beaten out of the town by the country-people, who poured in upon us in huge numbers; so that we were forced to retreat unto our boats, fighting our way through above 1000 men who were gathered against us; this was the hardest shock we had in all the South Sea. Captain Watling, our Commander-in-chief, was here killed; through whose ill-conduct, as it was thought, this misfortune happened unto us. For, had he assaulted the fort in time, before the people and soldiers that ran out of the town were got into it, we had undoubtedly carried all before us. But he trifled away his time in giving quarter and taking prisoners upon the breastworks, till at last we had more prisoners than we could command. We placed some of these prisoners before the front of our men, when we assaulted the castle, just as Sir Henry Morgan did the nuns and friars at Porto Bello, but the Spaniards fired at them as well as at us. In a word, we lost here 40 men, nine of which were taken prisoners, being our surgeons and others, while they were dressing the wounded at the hospital; which loss of our surgeons increased our damage very much, and only 42 or 43 were left serviceable to fight our way through so many hundred of foot and horse unto our boats, we not losing one man by the way, though several were wounded: so much did we awe them with our fuzees, and so afraid were they to break in upon us, though we were almost three miles from our boats. This repulse we resented almost more than any other we ever sustained before, since here was more plate and gold than we could well carry away, by reason it is the embarcadero, or place where all the vast riches that are brought from the mountains of Potosy are shipped off for Panama, whence it goes into Spain. Now Captain Sharp was chosen again, his conduct being thought safer than any other man's, and they having had trial of another leader. Our surgeons we left behind had quarter from the enemy, they being able to do good service in that country; but our wounded men were all knocked on the head, as we understood afterwards. This misfortune fell to us on the 30th of January, being King Charles' Day, as I can remember by some tokens.[11]

A kindly and quiet man, Esquemeling, speaking ill of no one. The truth of the

[10] Esquemeling. *Op. cit.*, p. 266–268.

[11] Esquemeling. *Op. cit.*, p. 274–275.

matter we have from the account of Basil Ringrose[12] which is that at the retreat Captain Sharp would have brought off the surgeons "but that they had been drinking while we assaulted the fort, and thus would not come with us when they were called."

Later, Spanish prisoners told them that the men taken prisoners at Arica were brought to Callao "and very civilly entertained there by all sorts of people, but more especially by the women. That one of our surgeons, whom we suspected to be Mr. Bullock, was left behind, and remained still at Arica." Which shadowy picture is all that is left us of Mr. Bullock and his two nameless fellow surgeons, lying drunk among the wounded in the Pirates' Hospital in that Chilean Coast town, while Watling and his handful were assaulting the fort; still lying there, too drunk to come when called, when the vanquished buccaneers at the end of their hot and bloody day finally fought their way through the choking dust to the beach and to their boats. And at the last, when "examined" (i.e. tortured) by their captors, betraying their comrades by divulging their signals.

In the meanwhile those of the town examined our surgeons and other men whom they had made prisoners. These gave them our signs that we had left to our boats that were behind us, so that they immediately blew up two smokes, which were perceived by the canoes. This was the greatest of our dangers. For, had we not come at the instant that we did to the sea-side, our boats had been gone, they being already under sail, and we had inevitably perished every man. Thus we put off from the shore, and got on board about ten o'clock at night, having been involved in a continual and bloody fight with the enemy all that day long.[13]

A shameful memory, Mr. Bullock!

With this same expedition was Lionel Wafer, another surgeon, whose figure remains on that faded canvas as one of the gentlest, most whimsical and engaging. On the fate-

ful day at Arica, Wafer was left with the guards at the boats, as a subordinate, preparing salves and plasters for the wounded. When the survivors regained their ship the capture of his drunken superiors left him surgeon-in-chief of what remained of the expedition. They set sail, cruised down the coast and up again. Ill-feeling between the faction which had chosen Watling commander and the Sharp faction continued until April 17, 1681, when off the Isle of Plata (Sir Francis Drake's isle, where he had divided Peruvian plunder among his men by the bowlful) open dissension broke out again and the party split. Forty-seven men, Wafer and the navigator Dampier among them, with five negro slaves and three Indians, set out in open boats for the Isthmus of Darien. Wafer has left an account of this voyage which was originally published in 1699 on his return to London, and has been reprinted several times. An accessible edition, with valuable notes, is that of G. P. Winship.[14] Enough detail can be gathered from this book, and from other accounts of the time to make a fairly coherent picture of Wafer's life. Several moderns have tried their hand at his portrait. R. Scot Skirving[15] wrote an essay on him; Sir Frederick Treves mentions him.[16]

His own delineation and those of his contemporaries will remain the best. The poet John Masefield, in the appendix to his edition of Dampier's Voyages, gives so accurate and concise a sketch of Wafer that to paraphrase it would be an unfair subterfuge. I shall repeat it.

LIONEL WAFER

This writer seems to have passed his youth "at the Navan upon the Boyne, and about the Town of Virginia upon Lough Ranor in the Barony of Castle Raghen in the County of

[12] Esquemeling. *Op.cit.*, p. 406-409.

[13] Esquemeling. *Op. cit.*, p. 409.

[14] Wafer, L. A New Voyage and Discovery of the Isthmus of America, etc. Ed. by Winship, G. Cleveland, 1903.

[15] Skirving, R. S. *Med. J. Australia*, Sydney April 12, 1924, I, 358.

[16] Treves. In the Cradle of the Deep. Lond., 1908

Cavan, and also in the Highlands of Scotland." In a manuscript preserved in the British Museum [Addl. Mss. 33054], he writes as though Wales were his native country, and England the land of his adoption. His parents, or guardians, seem to have been roving people of no position.

Wafer's "first going abroad was in the Great Anne of London, . . . bound for Bantam . . . in the year 1677." He was then "very young" (say 15 or 16), and "in the Service of the Surgeon" as loblolly boy, or dresser. The Great Anne visited Bantam, then sailed to Jamby in Sumatra, and then returned to Bantam to complete her cargo. Wafer seems to have gone ashore at Bantam with the intention of deserting. The Great Anne sailed without him, and he "got a Passage home" aboard a ship called the Bombay. He arrived in England in 1679, stayed a month, and then sailed (as loblolly boy) in a ship bound to Jamaica. He had a brother in Jamaica, employed at Sir Thomas Modyford's plantation at the Angel's. This brother kept him for a while, and then set him up as a surgeon in Port Royal, "where I followed my Business of Surgery for some Months."

Captain Lynch, or Linch, and Captain Edmund Cook, "two Privateers who were going out from Port Royal," persuaded Wafer to join them, as Surgeon. They visited the coasts of Cartagena, and arrived at the Bastimentos, near Porto Bello, in the early spring of 1680, shortly after the second taking of Porto Bello by Sawkins, Coxon, and Sharp. It was here that Wafer first met with Dampier.

Wafer accompanied Edmund Cook upon the march over the Isthmus to the South Seas. He was cruising in the Pacific with Sharp and the other buccaneers aboard the Holy Trinity, until after the battle of Arica, when the company divided. He returned with Dampier's party across the Isthmus; but on "the 5th day of our Journey" his leg was scorched by an explosion of powder; so that he was forced to stay behind among the Indians, with two other buccaneers, who could walk no further. The three were joined soon afterwards by two other stragglers.

Wafer "lived some Months" among the Indians "who in a Manner ador'd him by reason of his skill in Physik and Phlebotomy." He lived, he says, "in great Splendour and Repute"; and he alone, of the five prisoners, was painted "in yellow, red and blue, very bright, and lovely" as a mark of special affection. Eventually the five men reached La Sounds Key, where Captain Tristian took them aboard his cruiser. Wafer sailed under Tristian (having Dampier as a shipmate) for some days, and then went with Dampier, under Captains Wright and Yanky, for a cruise in the West Indies. At Salt Tortuga the two privateers parted company. Dampier stayed with Wright, and Wafer went with Yanky to the "Isle of Ash," or Vacca. Here he left Yanky in order to sail with John Cook (another of Sharp's party who had returned with Dampier) in a newly captured Spanish ship. The French objected that Cook had no commission and that he had no right to command the prize. They plundered the English seamen aboard her and then turned them ashore. Captain Tristian, who happened to be in the anchorage, received "about 8 or 10 of these English: of which number Captain Cook was one, and Captain Davis another," and (we surmise) Lionel Wafer a third. These "8 or 10" waited till Tristian went ashore at Tortuga, and then ran away with his ship, carried her back to Vacca, picked up the rest of the crew, and went a-cruising in her. They took a wine ship, and a ship of eight guns called the Revenge, in which they came to Virginia "about 8 or 9 months after Mr. Dampier came thither" (April, 1683). They fitted up the Revenge as their cruiser, and set sail aboard her August 23, 1683, on the voyage to Sierra Leone (where they took and went aboard the Batchelor's Delight). Wafer, who was one of the chirurgeons of the party, seems to have had a merry time among the African natives, while the Batchelor's Delight refitted. He took part in the adventures in the South Seas with Cook, Davis and the others until August 27, 1687, when Davis and Swan parted company. Dampier stayed with Swan; but Wafer remained in the Batchelor's Delight, under Davis, with whom were Captains Knight and Harris. After visiting Cocos Island, "the Gallapogo's," and "several of the Islands and Coasts of Peru," this squadron took Huavra, Huacho and Pisco. Davis then cruised westward, sighting what may have been Easter Island in the late autumn of 1687. They called at Juan Fernandez (where four men "would needs stay behind") and then sailed round the Horn on their way home. Near the Caribbee Islands, Wafer, Davis and others went aboard a Barbadoes sloop, and sailed in her up the Delaware to Philadelphia, where they arrived in May, 1688. One gathers that they settled in America, at Point Comfort, Va. "But meeting with some Troubles, after a 3 Years' Residence," Wafer returned to England (in the year 1690). The "Troubles" were a charge of piracy, which involved the whole party, and very nearly sent them to the gallows. Their booty (mostly silver) was taken from them, and they were forced to leave the colony; but, after several months in Newgate, in London, they were released (1691) and managed to win back the greater part of their spoil. Wafer was in London in 1697; for he then gave evidence before the Board of Trade and Plantations, concerning the settlement of the Isthmus of Darien. In 1699 he published his "New Voyage and Description," which he dedicated to the Earl of Romney. In or about the year 1700 he drew up a secret memorandum on places fit for settlement in the South Seas. This was done at the instance of the Duke of Marlborough, to whom (in 1704) the second edition of Wafer's book was dedicated. Wafer is said to have died in 1705. He is sometimes spoken of as De la Wafer.[17]

Whatever opinion Wafer himself may have had of the man, posterity has reason to be grateful to the "careless fellow" who scorched our jolly Keltic chirurgeon's knee and robbed him of his jolliness for a time. It was this accident that kept him behind his companions and made him fall into the hands of the Darien Indians and gave us one of the most entertaining of journals.

It was the 5th Day of our Journey when this Accident befel me; being also the 5th of May, in the Year 1681. I was sitting on the ground near one of our Men, who was drying of Gunpowder in a Silver Plate: But not managing it as he should, it blew up, and scorch'd my Knee to that Degree, that the Bone was left bare, the Flesh being torn away, and my Thigh burnt for a great way above it. I applied to it immediately such Remedies as I had in my Knapsack: And being unwilling to be left behind by my Companions, I made hard shift to jog on, and bear them Company for a few Days; during which our Slaves ran away from us, and among them a Negro whom the Company had allow'd me for my particular Attendant, to carry my Medi-

cines. He took them away with him, together with the rest of my Things, and thereby left me deprived of wherewithal to dress my Sore; insomuch that my Pain increasing upon me, and being not able to trudge it further through Rivers and Woods, I took leave of my Company, and set up my Rest among the Darien Indians.

This was on the 10th Day; and there staid with me Mr. Richard Gopson, who had served an Apprenticeship to a Druggist in London. He was an ingenious Man, and a good Scholar; and had with him a Greek Testament which he frequently read, and would translate extempore into English to such of the Company as were dispos'd to hear him. Another who staid behind with me was John Hingson, Mariner: They were both so fatigued with the Journey, that they could go no further. There had been an Order made among us at our first Landing, to kill any who should flag in the Journey: But this was made only to terrify any from loitering, and being taken by the Spaniards; who by Tortures might extort from them a Discovery of our March. But this rigorous Order was not executed; but the Company took a very kind Leave both of these, and of me. . . .

Being now forc'd to stay among them, and having no means to alleviate the Anguish of my Wound, the Indians undertook to cure me; and apply'd to my Knee some Herbs, which they first chew'd in their Mouths to the consistency of a Paste, and putting it on a Plantain-Leaf, laid it upon the Sore. This proved so effectual, that in about 20 Days use of this Poultess, which they applied fresh every Day, I was perfectly cured; except only a Weakness in that Knee, which remained long after, and a Benumbness which I sometimes find in it to this Day. Yet they were not altogether so kind in other respects; for some of them look'd on us very scurvily throwing green Plantains to us, as we sat cringing and shivering, as you would Bones to a Dog.[18]

With Wafer were four other men. One more was drowned while swimming a river with a line about his neck, "the stream running very swift and the man having three hundred dollars at his back, was carried down, and never seen more by us." His companions roaming the woods to rejoin Wafer "saw him lie dead on the

[17] Masefield, J. Dampier's Voyages. 1, 536–538.

[18] Wafer, *Op. cit.*, p. 36–39.

Shore which the Floods were gone off from, with the Rope twisted about him, and his Mony at his Neck; but they were so fatigued, they car'd not to meddle with it."[19] Wafer apologized for the Indians' harsh treatment:

Not that they were naturally inclin'd to use us thus roughly for they are generally a kind and free-hearted People; but they had taken some particular Offence, upon the account of our Friends who left us, who had in a manner awed the Indian Guides they took with them for the remainder of their Journey, and made them go with them very much against their Wills.[20]

The smaller party of stragglers found a Spanish-speaking Indian who brought them food by stealth, and kept them while their captors, fearful that the two Indians forced by Dampier and the rest of the party to act as guides might have come to harm, debated whether to kill them or not.

But it so hapned that Lacenta, their Chief, passing that way, dissuaded them from that Cruelty, and proposed to them to send us down towards the North-side, and two Indians with us, who might inform themselves from the Indians near the Coast, what was become of the Guides. They readily hearken'd to this Proposal and immediately chose two Men to conduct us to the North-side.[21]

They kept their guides for three days, when their scanty provision being spent, these returned home again and left Wafer and his companions to shift for themselves. Starving, they floundered about in the rainy woods and camped by swollen streams for eight days.

The Night was still very dark, but only when the flashes of Lightning came: Which made it so dreadful and terrible, that I forgot my Hunger, and was wholly taken up with praying to God to spare my Life. While I was Praying and Meditating thus on my sad Condition, I saw the Morning Star appear, by which I knew that Day was at hand: This cheared my drooping Spirits, and in less than half an hour the Day began to dawn, the Rain and Lightning ceas'd and the Waters abated.[22]

After many mishaps they turned about and rejoined the Indians at the same camp from which they had set out. They were well received; the two Indian guides had returned safely and had been well used.

We had not been long here before an Occurence happen'd, which tended much to the increasing the good Opinion Lacenta and his People had conceiv'd of us, and brought me into particular Esteem with them.

It so happen'd, that one of Lacenta's Wives being indisposed, was to be let Blood; which the Indians perform in this manner: The Patient is seated on a Stone in the River, and one with a small Bow shoots little Arrows into the naked Body of the Patient, up and down; shooting them as fast as he can, and not missing any part. But the Arrows are gaged, so that they penetrate no farther than we generally thrust our Lancets: And if by chance they hit a Vein which is full of Wind, and the Blood spurts out a little, they will leap and skip about, shewing many Antick Gestures, by way of rejoycing and triumph.

I was by while this was performing on Lacenta's Lady: And perceiving their Ignorance, told Lacenta, That if he pleased I would shew him a better way, without putting the Patient to so much Torment. Let me see, says he; and at his Command, I bound up her Arm with a piece of Bark, and with my Lancet breathed a Vein: But this rash attempt had like to have cost me my Life. For Lacenta seeing the Blood issue out in a Stream, which us'd to come only drop by drop, got hold of his Lance, and swore by his Tooth that if she did otherwise than well, he would have my Heart's Blood. I was not moved, but desired him to be patient, and I drew off about 12 Ounces, and bound up her Arm, and desired she might rest till the next Day: By which means the Fever abated, and she had not another Fit. This gained me so much Reputation, that Lacenta came to me, and before all his Attendants, bowed, and kiss'd my Hand. Then the rest came thick about me, and some kissed my Hand, others my Knee, and some my Foot: After which I was taken up into a Hammock,

19 Wafer, p. 41.
20 Wafer, p. 40.
21 Wafer, p. 42.

22 Wafer, p. 48.

and carried on Men's Shoulders, Lacenta himself making a Speech in my Praise, and commending me as much Superior to any of their Doctors. Thus I was carried from Plantation to Plantation, and lived in great Splendor and Repute, administering both Physick and Phlebotomy to those that wanted. For tho' I lost my Salves and Plaisters, when the Negro ran away with my Knapsack, yet I preserv'd a Box of Instruments, and a few Medicaments wrapt up in an Oil-Cloth, by having them in my Pocket, where I generally carried them.

I lived thus for some Months among the Indians, who in a manner ador'd me . . ."[23]

After this Wafer had as hard a time in getting away from his new friends as he had had in first ingratiating himself with them. Finally he pictured to Lacenta the great advantages of English hunting dogs and offered to bring him a few from England if he would but allow him to go and get them.

Lacenta . . . demurred at this Motion a while; but at length he swore by his Tooth, laying his Fingers on it, That I should have my Liberty and for my Sake the other four with me; provided I would promise and swear by my Tooth, that I would return and live among them; for he had made me a promise of his Daughter in Marriage, but she was not then marriageable. I accepted of the Conditions: and he further promised, that at my return he would do for me beyond my Expectation.[24]

So under the convoy of seven lusty fellows, Wafer and his four companions made their way to the coast, where arriving they found the first part of the expedition lying with two ships.

We went aboard the English Sloop, and our Indian Friends with us, and were received with a very hearty welcome. The four English Men with me were presently known and caress'd by the Ships Crew; but I sat a while cringing upon my Hams among the Indians, after their Fashion, painted as they were, and all naked but only about the Waist, and with my Nosepiece (of which more hereafter) hanging over my Mouth. I was willing to try if they would know me in this Disguise; and 'twas the better part of

an Hour before one of the Crew, looking more narrowly upon me, cry'd out, Here's our Doctor; and immediately they all congratulated my Arrival among them. I did what I could presently to wash off my Paint, but 'twas near a Month before I could get tolerably rid of it, having had my Skin so long stain'd with it, and the Pigment dried on in the Sun: And when it did come off, 'twas usually with the peeling off of Skin and all. As for Mr. Gopson, tho' we brought him alive to the Ship, yet he did not recover his Fatigues, and his drenching in the Water, but having languish'd aboard about three Days, he died there at La Sound's Key.[25]

Thus ends the account of his travels over the Isthmus. In the succeeding chapters of his journal he relates of Isthmian animals, trees and plants, of the Indians and their customs, and adds a short vocabulary of their language.

He evidently does not wish his book to compete with or duplicate the journal of his old shipmate Dampier, published a few years before. He confines his account to territory which he explored apart from Dampier; he adds a final chapter on his travels with Captain Davis in the Batchelor's Delight, Dampier having gone with Captain Swan in the Cygnet.

We left them in the Harbour of Realeja, when we set out Aug. 27, 1685, with three other Vessels in our Company. But our Men growing very sick when we were got out to Sea, we soon put into the Gulph of Amapalla. There we lay several Weeks at a small Island, on which we built Huts for our sick Men, whom we put ashore. In our 4 small Ships, we had then above 130 sick of the Spotted Fever, many of whom died: Yet tho' I attended them every Day, I thank God I escap'd the Infection.[26]

They travelled up and down the Chilian and Peruvian Coast and took various towns. At Vermejo, seeking for water, they landed at a sandy Bay, where they found the beach "covered with the Bodies of Men, Women, and Children; which lay so thick, that a Man might, if he would, have walked half a Mile, and never trod a step off a dead

[23] Wafer, p. 54–55.
[24] Wafer, p. 58.

[25] Wafer, p. 64–65.
[26] Wafer, p. 173.

human Body. These Bodies, to appearance, seem'd as if they had not been above a Week dead; but if you handled them, they prov'd as dry and light as a Spunge or piece of Cork."[27]

They asked an old Indian how these bodies came there. In his father's time, the Indian said, the soil had been well cultivated and fruitful, but when the Spaniards came and blocked up and laid siege to the city, the Indians, rather than lie at the Spaniards' mercy, dug holes in the sand and buried themselves alive.

The Men as they now lie, have with them their broken Bows; and the Women their Spinning-wheels, and Distaffs with Cotton-yarn upon them. Of these dead Bodies I brought on board a Boy of about 9 or 10 Years of Age, with an intent to bring him home for England: But was frustrated of my purpose by the Sailors; who having a foolish Conceit, that the Compass would not traverse aright, so long as any dead Body was on board, threw him overboard, to my great Vexation.[28]

They rounded the Horn in a great storm, coasted along Brazil and had made the Caribbee Islands when they heard of King James' pardon to the buccaneers. Wafer and some others took advantage of it and sailed up the Delaware to Philadelphia. From here they carted their "Chests and other Goods" overland to Chesapeake Bay, thinking to settle on the James River in Virginia. "But meeting with some Troubles, after a three years residence there, I came home for England, in the year 1690." The troubles, as Masefield says, were charges of piracy. Perhaps their "Chests and other Goods" had something to do with them.

Thus ends Wafer's journal. A kindly, helpful, jolly, whimsical man: seeing the best in his fellows, condoning their faults, speaking ill of no one; ready at a prank and masquerading as an Indian in paint and feathers when he rejoins his ship after all his mishaps—a true Gael; a good naturalist and observer, writing sensibly and entertainingly of llamas and ostriches and other beasts, birds and plants; a generous and loyal man, yielding in his writings to his difficult and cantankerous shipmate Dampier; trusty and helpful, nursing 130 sick with spotted fever and thanking God he escaped the infection; a proper good doctor to help a company of rovers through unknown tropical forests, sickness and battles with man and Nature.

We owe most of our knowledge of the buccaneers to the excellent historian Esquemeling, another surgeon and colleague: an uncommonly well-balanced and unimpassioned person, an ideal narrator. Of his own life he has left us but a few flimsy threads, nor do we find mention of him in other writers of the time. We know next to nothing of his career, or where and how he lived and died, but his character we can fill in from his writings. "The Buccaneers of America: a True Account of the most remarkable Assaults committed of late years upon the coast of the West Indies by the Buccaneers of Jamaica and Tortuga, both English and French wherein are contained more especially the unparalleled Exploits of Sir Henry Morgan, our English Jamaican Hero, who sacked Porto Bello, burnt Panama, etc.

"Written originally in Dutch by John Esquemeling one of the Buccaneers who was present at these tragedies.

"Translated into Spanish by Alonso de Bonne-Maison, M.D., etc. Now faithfully rendered into English with Facsimiles of all the original Engravings, Maps, etc. Translation of 1684-5."

This book was originally written in Dutch and published in Amsterdam in 1678 under the title of "De Americaensche Zeerovers." It was soon translated into English and passed through several editions, many of them amended and changed by the publisher to save the renown of some of the more popular English heroes, especially Sir Henry Morgan. A new edition by Wm. Swan Stallybrass has been issued in the Broadway translations.[29]

---

[27] Wafer, p. 186.
[28] Wafer, p. 187.

[29] Lond. and N. Y.

Esquemeling set sail, he says, from Havre-de-Grace in France in a ship called the St. John, on the second of May, 1666, and landed at Tortuga, near Haiti, on the seventh of July of the same year. Tortuga had been captured from the Spanish by French buccaneers, and a governor had been sent them by the governor of the French colony of St. Christopher. In 1664 this governor was dispossessed by the French West India Company who sent a governor of their own, a Monsieur Ogeron. Under charter of the French government the Company thought to have a monopoly of trade with the hunters, buccaneers and planters, inhabitants of the island, and also to drive trade with the Spanish, as the Dutch did at Curaçao. This design was a failure, for the factors of the Company soon found that they could not "recover either moneys or returns from these people." They sent out armed men and tried to make their collections by force, a futile scheme.

And hereupon the Company recalled their factors, giving them orders to sell all that was their own in the said plantation, both the servants belonging to the Company (which were sold, some for 20, others for 30, pieces-of-eight), as also all other merchandizes and properties which they had there. With this resolution all their designs fell to the ground.

In this occasion I was also sold, as being a servant under the said Company, in whose service I came out of France. But my fortune was very bad, for I fell into the hands of the most cruel tyrant and perfidious man that ever was born of woman, who was then Governor, or rather Lieutenant-General, of that island. This man treated me with all the hard usages imaginable, yea, with that of hunger, with which I thought to have perished inevitably. Withal he was willing to let me buy my freedom and liberty, but not under the rate of 300 pieces-of-eight, I not being master of one, at that time, in the whole world. At last through the manifold miseries I endured, as also affliction of mind, I was thrown into a dangerous fit of sickness. This misfortune, being added to the rest of my calamities, was the cause of my happiness. For my wicked master, seeing my condition,

began to fear lest he should lose his moneys with my life. Hereupon he sold me the second time to a surgeon for the price of 70 pieces-of-eight. Being in the hands of this second master, I began soon after to recover my health through the good usage I had received from him as being much more humane and civil than that of my first patron. He gave me both clothes and very good food, and after that I had served him but one year he offered me my liberty, with only this condition, that I should pay him 100-pieces-of-eight when I was in a capacity of wealth so to do. Which kind proposal of his I could not choose but accept with infinite joy and gratitude of mind.

Being now at liberty, though like unto Adam when he was first created by the hands of his Maker—that is, naked and destitute of all human necessaries, nor knowing how to get my living—I determined to enter into the wicked order of the Pirates, or Robbers at Sea. Into this Society I was received with common consent both of the superior and vulgar sort, and among them I continued until the year 1672. Having assisted them in all their designs and attempts, and served them in many notable exploits of which hereafter I shall give the reader a true account, I returned to my own native country.[30]

This is all we have of his personal history. His book is incomparable. It is the sole record of older and later buccaneers, of Frenchmen and Portuguese of an unthinkable savagery; of L'Olonnois, who tore the living heart from his Spanish victim's breast and gnawed at it in his rage; of the later race of Mansvelt, Sir Henry Morgan, Sawkins, Harris and Cook, Wafer's captains and comrades. It is a faithful and minute chronicle of buccaneer customs, codes and government; it records the bloodiest and most ferocious ravages with the same Flemish tranquillity with which it recounts the habits of West Indian birds and fishes; it breathes withal a steady Lutheran spirit of Christianity. This peaceful Flemish surgeon-apprentice found no pleasure in the savagery of his French shipmates, but he left us an extraordinary chronicle of them.

[30] Esquemeling. *Op. cit.*, p. 21–22.

He was with Morgan in his sack of Panama; he was deserted by him later, when Morgan stole off with the booty, cheating his fellow buccaneers of their legitimate shares.

What became of him or where he died we do not know. He has but the two paragraphs quoted above of himself, others mention him only to quote from his writings. His must have been a gentle, kindly and modest nature. Even those who injured him he seeks to excuse.

These two buccaneers, Wafer and Esquemeling, have been preserved to us as historians rather than surgeons. Neither appears to have had a degree, both learned their professions not at schools but by apprenticeship to surgeons whose names are lost to us. Unless perhaps the tipsy Mr. Bullock was Wafer's master.

A third seafaring doctor's name is preserved in a powder rather than by his navigations. And justly so, for the powder has stood the test of time.

Osler has written a delightful essay on this man: I shall refer you to it[31] and spare you lengthy detail concerning Dr. Dover, sea rover and originator of the pulv. ipecac. et opii comp. A squabbling, irascible, Paracelsian character, with considerable of the mountebank even for those eighteenth century days; author of a medical manual for laymen; always ready to pick a quarrel with his colleagues; an opinionated stubborn man. Yet let us given him his due: his love of adventure was such that at the age of forty-eight he gave up his practice in Bristol, fitted out a privateering expedition and set out on it himself. His book is entitled "The Ancient Physician's Legacy to his Country, Being what he has collected in Forty-Nine Years' Practice: or an Account of the several Diseases incident to Mankind, in so plain a Manner, that any Person may know the Nature of his own Distemper, and the several Remedies proper for it, wherein the extraordinary Effects of Mercury are

more particularly consider'd. Design'd for the Use of all Private Families. By Thomas Dovar, M.D. with Remarks on the Whole by a Learned Physician. To which is added (being a proper Supplement to the Work) a New Translation of a Treatise of Mercury, and the Wonderful Cures performed by it; written by the Learned Belloste, Author of the Hospital Surgeon. With a complea't Index to the whole. London. Printed for the Relict of the late R. Bradly. 1733."

The old man (he was seventy-two or seventy-three when he wrote the book) held no mean opinion of himself:

If travelling be necessary to make an accomplished Physician, I am very sure that I have travelled more than all the Physicians in Great-Britain put together.

But I am going a little out of my Way, and shall therefore return to what I at first proposed; wherein, if I fall short, I shall yet please myself in my sincere Design of being beneficial to Mankind. All I desire of those who find fault with my Performance, is to produce a better in its Room.[32]

He was no timid therapeutist:

When we took the two Cities of Guaiaquil, under the Line, in the South-Sea it happened, that not long before the Plague had raged amongst them. For our better Security therefore, and keeping our People together, we lay in their Churches; and likewise brought thither the Plunder of the Cities: We were very much annoyed with the Smell of dead Bodies. These Bodies could hardly be said to be buried; for the Spaniards abroad use no Coffins, but throw several dead Bodies one upon another; with only a Draw-Board over them; so that 'tis no Wonder we received the Infection.

In a very few Days after we got on Board, one of the Surgeons came to me to acquaint me, that several of my Men were taken after a so violent Manner with the Langour of Spirits, that they were not able to move. I immediately went among them, and to my great Surprise soon discerned what was the Matter. In less than forty-eight Hours we had in our several Ships one hundred and eighty Men in this miserable Condition.

[31] Osler, Sir W. An Alabama Student and Other Biographical Essays. Oxford, 1908.

[32] Dover, p. 7–8.

I ordered the Surgeons to bleed them in both Arms, and to go round to them all, with Command to leave them bleeding till all were blooded, and then come and tie them up in their Turns. They lay bleeding and fainting, so long, that I could not conceive they could lose less than an hundred Ounces each Man.

. . . So that notwithstanding we had one hundred and eighty odd down in this most fatal Distemper, yet we lost no more than seven or eight; and even these owed their Deaths to the strong Liquors which their Mess-Mates procured for them.

They had all Spots, which in the great Plague they call Tokens; few or none of the Spaniards escaped Death that had them; but my People had them, and Buboes too.

Now if we had had Recourse to Alexipharmicks, such as Venice Treacle, Diascordium, Mithridate, and such like good-for-nothing Compositions, or the most celebrated Gascoin's Powder, or Bezoar, I make no Question at all, considering the Heat of the Climate, but we had lost every man.[33]

This passage called down the gibe that Osler mentions:

I think the Doctor had much better left out his Bravado of having taken two cities by storm, unless he thinks it an honour to a Physician to kill and slay, and after to plunder the Innocent, those who never wronged him, and to carry off the spoil; a good prelude, this, to the blood shed after among his own men.[34]

The doctor himself considered the copious use of native quicksilver as his chief legacy. As addenda to his book there are a number of testimonials: thus his obliged humble servant Benj. Benson, who suffered from scorbutic humours and a white scurf on the hands in the spring, writes from Piccadilly on May 10, 1739, to say that he had taken in all some five pounds of the crude mercury and believed it to be "the best Remedy in obstinate chronick Diseases, and nothing more pleasant and agreeable."

Dover's medical portrait is scarcely a venerable one: he had, as Osler says, the wit to compound a good powder, but he apparently held it in no particular esteem. He thought more highly of more violent remedies; he lacked the genius of a Paracelsus or even common sense; no foundation of usefulness underlay his mountebankery.

Let us leave Dr. Dover. Captain Dover is more entertaining..

The expedition in which he sailed from Bristol was well financed, well equipped and well planned. And it was no fault, but rather the effect of wisdom, forethought and cautiousness, if it lacked some of the savor of romance and adventure that fired the expeditions of the earlier buccaneers. The venture was unusually successful: far from returning bankrupt, as that incomparable naturalist, scientist and navigator, but mighty poor pirate Dampier had, it brought back a booty of £170,000.

It was financed by Bristol men, among them Dr. Dover; it was commanded by Captain Woodes-Rogers, afterward governor of the Bahamas, than whom there was no better commander. With them sailed Dampier, whose knowledge of the art of navigation, of winds, tides and currents, and of the geography of the South Seas was unequalled. The doctor took the title of captain and sailed as third in command; "as owner of a very considerable share of both vessels, he was President of the Council and had a double voice in the deliberations." (Osler.) In October, 1701, they sailed from Bristol for the South Seas (the Pacific) in two ships, the Duke and Duchess.

On February 1, 1710, they sighted the Island of Juan Fernandez off the Chilean coast; the next day Captain Dover, with a Mr. Fry and six men, went ashore and discovered Alexander Selkirk, the original of Robinson Crusoe, a man who had been left on the Island four and a half years before by Captain Stradling of the Cinque-Portes. Dampier had sailed in this vessel and had known the man. I shall not quote Captain Woodes-Rogers' account of this discovery. Osler repeats it in full.

---

[33] Dover, p. 67–69.
[34] Turner, D. Quoted by Osler, Sir W. *Johns Hopkins Hosp. Bull.*, Balt., 1896, VII, 5.

Here is adventure enough to justify remembering this old Bristol privateer-doctor. But he did not only this. Later he led an assault on Guayaquil and captured it; and later still he was given command of a prize-ship, renamed the Batchelor, now truly Captain Dover. Where he learned his navigation does not appear, but he must have been a competent commander to have held an independent position in a company that included Captain Woodes-Rogers and Dampier.

Your memory therefore is assured, Captain Dover, even though your powder and quicksilver, Dr. Dover, be forgotten. Robinson Crusoe, Defoe and Captain Woodes-Rogers have saved you.

Thomas Lodge, sea rover and poet, was not strictly a buccaneer doctor. He studied medicine later, after he left the sea. He was born about 1557; his father was Sir Thomas Lodge, grocer and Lord Mayor of London in 1563. The Encyclopedia Brittanica has an essay on him, ready to every man's hand. He was educated at the Merchant Tailors' School and at Trinity College, Oxford. Between 1584-1590 he engaged in more than one free-booting expedition to the Spanish Main. On August 26, 1591, he sailed from Plymouth for Brazil with Sir Thomas Cavendish in the galleon Desire. The tale of the expedition is full of misery. They took the town of Santos while the people were at Mass but got nothing.

Such was the negligence of our governor master Cocke, that the Indians were suffered to carry out of the towne whatsoever they would in open viewe, and no man did controll them: and the next day after wee had wonne the towne, our prisoners were all set at libertie, onely foure poore olde men were kept as pawnes to supply our wants. Thus in three dayes the towne that was able to furnish such another Fleete with all kinde of necessaries, was left unto us nakedly bare, without people and provision. Eight or tenne dayes after master Candish himselfe came thither, where hee remained untill the 22. of January, seeking by intreatie to have that, whereof we were once possessed.

But in conclusion wee departed out of the towne through extreme want of victuall, not being able any longer to live there, and were glad to receive a few canisters or baskets of Cassavi meale; so that in every condition wee went worse furnished from the towne, then when wee came unto it. The 22. of January we departed from Santos, and burnt Sant Vincent to the ground. The 24. we set saile, shaping our course for the Streights of Magellan.[35]

At Santos Lodge took up his quarters with some others of the English in the Jesuit College, and spent five weeks there among the books in the Father's library. From March until December they cruised about Patagonia and the Straits of Magellan, struggling with hunger, disease and mutiny:

In the which time wee indured extreme stormes, with perpetual snow, where many of our men died with cursed famine, and miserable cold, not having wherewith to cover their bodies, nor to fill their bellies, but living by muskles, water, and weeds of the sea, with a small reliefe of the ships store in meale sometimes. And all the sicke men in the Galeon were most uncharitably put a shore into the woods in the snowe, raine, and cold, when men of good health could scarcely indure it, where they ended their lives in the highest degree of misery, master Candish all this while being abord the Desire.[36]

Here the unruffled poet wrote his romance "Marguerite of America."

The expedition reached Ireland June 11, 1593. They had victualled their ship with dried penguins; on the return voyage, as they came "neere unto the sun, our dried Penguins began to corrupt, and there bred in them a most lothsome & ugly worme of an inch long."

This worme did so mightily increase, and devoure our victuals, that there was in reason no hope how we should avoide famine; but be devoured of these wicked creatures: there was nothing that they did not devour, only yron excepted: our clothes, boots, shooes, hats, shirts, stockings: and for the ship they did so eat the timbers, as that we greatly feared they would

[35] Hakluyt. Everyman Ed., VIII, 289-290.
[36] Hakluyt. VIII, 291.

undoe us, by gnawing through the ships side. Great was the care and diligence of our captain, master, and company to consume these vermine, but the more we laboured to kill them, the more they increased; so that at the last we could not sleepe for them, but they would eate our flesh, and bite like Mosquitos. In this wofull case, after we had passed the Equinoctiall toward the North, our men began to fall sick of such a monstrous disease, as I thinke the like was never hearde of: for in their ankles it began to swell; from thence in two daies it would be in their breasts, so that they could not draw their breath, and then fell into their cods; and their cods and yardes did swell most grievously, and most dreadfully to behold, so that they could neither stand, lie, nor goe. Whereupon our men grew mad with griefe. Our Captain with extreme anguish of his soule, was in such wofull case, that he desired only a speedie end, and though he were scarce able to speak for sorrow, yet he perswaded them to patience, and to give God thanks, & like dutifull children to accept of his chastisement. For all this divers grew raging mad, & some died in most lothsome & furious paine. It were incredible to write our misery as it was: there was no man in perfect health, but the captain & one boy. The master being a man of good spirit with extreme labour bore out his griefe, so that it grew not upon him. To be short, all our men died except 16, of which there were but 5 able to moove. The captaine was in good health, the master indifferent, captaine Cotton and my selfe swolne and short winded, yet better than the rest that were sicke, and one boy in health: upon us 5 only the labour of the ship did stand. The captaine and master, as occasion served, would take in, and heave out the top-sailes, the master onely attended on the sprit-saile, and all of us at the capstan without sheats and tacks. In fine our miserie and weaknesse was so great, that we could not take in, nor heave out a saile: so our top-saile and sprit-sailes were torne all in pieces by the weather. The master and captaine taking their turnes at the helme, were mightily distressed and monstrously grieved with the most wofull lamentation of our sick men. Thus as lost wanderers upon the sea, the 11 of June 1593, it pleased God that we arrived at Bearhaven in Ireland, and there ran the ship on shore.[37]

[37] Hakluyt. VIII, 310–311.

This voyage seems to have turned the venturous poet from sailoring to the gentler business of medicine. He went to Avignon where he graduated in 1600, at the age of forty. He wrote a treatise on the plague (1603) and died of this disease in 1625, aged sixty-eight, medicine having brought him more success than had the sea.

Beside Lodge and Dover, and the two rover surgeons Wafer and Esquemeling, whose works of travel have kept their names alive, there is a host of others concerning whose lives we have to look to contemporary writings. Some of them hold the buccaneer stage long enough to provoke compassion, admiration, or a smile; more of them flit by, dim names, or nameless shadows. Many of them are mentioned in connection with various diseases and scourges that beset the fleets; others have come down to us for deeds of piracy or daring; others, sad to say, for their faults. The names are many: one might without much trouble list them in a medico-piratical encyclopedia, as Philip Gosse has done for the buccaneers.

Among the early ones is Nicholas Millechap, Sir Walter Raleigh's surgeon on his first voyage to Guiana in the Lion's Whelp (1595). "Our chirurgeon, Nicholas Millechap, brought me a kind of stones like sapphires; what they may prove I know not," he says.

Sir Walter Raleigh lost the surgeon of his unfortunate second voyage while off the Island of Santiago (Cape Verde Islands). "Monday being Michaelmas Day (September 29, 1617), then died our Master Surgeon, Mr. Nubal, to our great loss; . . . and we had 60 men sick, and all mine own servants amongst them, that I had none of mine own but my pages to serve me."

Of Sir Francis Drake's surgeons I can find but little. His expeditions were conducted with much secrecy and intrigue. The accounts of the deeds of this most glorious of all sea rovers are fragmentary and contradictory. Soon after his death his adventures shone with a halo of myth, like those of King Arthur, and the lesser lights of his medical men were put out by the effulgence of the sun about which their orbits revolved. On his glorious third voyage to the Spanish Main (1572), in which he first viewed the Pacific, he carried with him a doctor who seems not to have been a "great proficient" in his art (Masefield). While off the Isthmus of Panama at Fort Diego, a day or two after New Year of 1573, "half a score of our Company fell down sick together, and the most of them died within two or three days." They called the sickness a calenture and attributed it to the sudden change from cold to heat or to the brackish water they took on board, more likely the latter. Thirty of the men were down with it at one time; among the dead was Joseph Drake, brother of Sir Francis, "who died in our Captain's arms." Drake, to stop the panic among his men and "that the cause of the disease might be better discerned, and consequently remedied" had the surgeon open his brother's corpse. The surgeon "found his liver swollen, his heart as it were sodden, and his gut all fair." "This was the first and last experiment that our Captain made of anatomy in this voyage." The surgeon who made the examination "overlived him not past four days," a fact which, Masefield maliciously but perhaps not untruthfully adds, very possibly saved the lives of half the company.

He had had the sickness at its first beginning among them, but had recovered. He died, we are told, "of an overbold practice which he would needs make upon himself, by receiving an overstrong purgation of his own device, after which taken he never spake; nor his Boy recovered the health which he lost by tasting it, till he saw England." He seems to have taken the draught directly after the operation, as a remedy against infection from the corpse. The boy, who, perhaps, acted as assistant at the operation, may have thought it necessary to drink his master's heeltaps by way of safeguard.[38]

His nephew and namesake's description of his (fifth) great voyage around the

[38] Masefield. *Op. cit.*, p. 42.

world, entitled "The World Encompassed" (Hakluyt Society's Publications) contains a note on Drake's doctors. It was on this voyage that Drake, continuing up the West Coast of America, discovered California, naming it New Albion. At Drake's Bay near Bolinas he landed and nailing to a tree a leaden tablet with the name of Queen Elizabeth scratched on it, took possession for his sovereign.

The doctors are mentioned in the description of an affray on an island off the Chilean Coast, after the Golden Hind had weathered the Straits of Magellan. The note reads:

The rest, being nine persons in the boat were deadly wounded in divers parts of their bodies, if God almost miraculously had not given cure to the same. For our chief surgeon being dead and the other absent by the losse of our Vice-Admirall, and having none left us but a boy, whose good will was more than any skill hee had, wee were little better than altogether destitute of such cunning and helpes as so grievous a state of so many wounded bodies did require.[39]

On Drake's last voyage his chief surgeon was James Wood. Touching at the Canary Isles on this voyage, the surgeon of one of the fleet's ships, the Solomon, went up a hill with six or seven companions to fetch water. They were set upon by herdsmen with staves and the captain and three or four of the party were killed; the surgeon was taken prisoner "who disclosed our pretended voyage as much as in him lay; so as the Viceroy sent a caravel of adviso into the Indies, with all such places as wee did pretend to goe to."

Immediately upon reaching the West Indies, dysentery broke out among them. The vice-admiral, Sir John Hawkins, was among the first to die of it. The chief surgeon Wood died January 27, 1596 off Puerto Bello; Drake followed him the next day and was buried on an island off the coast of Panama, a fit resting place for the greatest of captains of the sea.

[39] Drake, F. The World Encompassed. Pub. by Hakluyt Soc., p. 98.

With the later rovers, the real buccaneers, there sailed a host of surgeons, named and nameless; some rascals, some jolly figures, some serious minded men, with an eye to the main chance. A diverting trail to follow.

Among the nameless ones is the surgeon of Pierre-le-Grand, pioneer buccaneer. Pierre made sure that there was to be no retreat (*vid. supra*) when his band swarmed aboard the Spanish galleon; he entrusted the task of scuttling his abandoned boat to his medico, whose dependability with the augur may have exceeded his courage.

Another nameless one was the surgeon of M. Ogeron, governor of Tortuga. In 1673, during the war between France and Holland, M. Ogeron joined forces with a French fleet with the intention of proceeding against the Dutch West Indies. They sailed for Curaçao, but were shipwrecked on the shores of Porto Rico, many of them were killed by the Spaniards and the rest taken prisoners, M. Ogeron among them. "He kept himself very close to all the features and mimical actions that might become any innocent fool. Upon this account he was not tied like the rest of his companions, but let loose, to serve the divertisement and laughter of the common soldiers."

It happened there was found among the French Pirates a certain surgeon, who had done some remarkable services to the Spaniards. In consideration of these merits, he was unbound and set at liberty, to go freely up and down, even as Monsieur Ogeron did. Unto this surgeon Monsieur Ogeron, having a fit opportunity thereunto, declared his resolution of hazarding his life to attempt an escape from the cruelty and hard usage of those enemies.[40]

Ogeron and his surgeon fled into the woods, and after many hardships built a canoe, with which they crossed to Haiti, landing in Samana. Here Ogeron "gave orders unto the surgeon to levy all the people he could possibly in those parts while he departed to revisit his government of Tortuga."[41]

[40] Esquemeling. *Op. cit.*, p. 244.
[41] Esquemeling. *Op. cit.*, p. 245.

He embarked the forces which his surgeon had gathered at Samana and again set out for Porto Rico. The Spaniards had been apprised of this new expedition; they laid an ambuscade and destroyed the greater part of the force. The remainder they took prisoners and transported them to Europe by degrees, in order to disperse them. Many of them, however, worked their way back to Tortuga again and undertook a new expedition against the Spanish and Dutch, this time with better success.

A serious-minded man, yet not untouched by human foibles nor even by the allurements of the female, was Mr. Herman Coppinger, surgeon and Dampier's companion on his first long voyage around the world. We first hear of him at the Island of Sal in the Cape Verdes, buying spurious ambergris.

We stay'd here 3 days; in which time one of these Portuguese offered to some of our Men a lump of Ambergreece in exchange for some Cloaths, desiring them to keep it secret, for he said if the Governor should know it he should be hanged. At length one Mr. Coppinger bought it for a small matter; yet I believe he gave more than it was worth. We had not a Man in the Ship that knew Ambergreece; but I have since seen it in other places, and therefore am certain it was not right. It was of a dark colour, like Sheeps Dung, and very soft, but of no smell, and possibly 'twas some of their Goats Dung.[42]

Thus was Mr. Coppinger at the outset of his travels still trusting and gullible. I doubt whether he would have been so ready later to buy goat's dung for ambergris as he was at the time of his sojourn among the primitive gold-brick men of the Cape Verde Isles.

His next appearance is more exciting. The voyage seems to have come to a long halt at Mindanao. The Filipino ladies (Pagalies), offered by the hospitable inhabitants (for a consideration) to the crew, were too much for the ship's discipline. Dampier's captain, Swan, spent all of his time ashore. The crew was mostly drunk (those that had

[42] Dampier, I, 101.

money); those that had none were quarrelsome and dissatisfied and wanted to go on. After seven months' delay a mutiny broke out. Captain Snow was ashore; the mutineers were aboard ready to sail.

Which would have been presently, if the Surgeon or his Mate had been aboard; but they were both ashore, and they thought it no Prudence to go to sea without a Surgeon: Therefore the next Morning they sent ashore one John Cookworthy, to hasten off either the Surgeon or his Mate, by pretending that one of the Men in the Night broke his Leg by falling into the Hold. The Surgeon told him that he intended to come aboard the next day with the Captain, and would not come before; but sent his Mate, Herman Coppinger.

This Man sometime before this, was sleeping at his Pagallies and a Snake twisted himself about his Neck; but afterwards went away without hurting him. In this Country it is usual to have the Snakes come into the Houses and into the Ships too; for we had several came aboard our Ship when we lay in the River. But to proceed, Herman Coppinger provided to go aboard; and the next day, being the time appointed for Captain Swan and all his Men to meet aboard, I went aboard with him, neither of us distrusted what was designing by those aboard, till we came thither. Then we found it was only a trick to get the Surgeon off; for now, having obtained their Desires, the Canoa was sent ashore again immediately, to desire as many as they could meet to come aboard; but not to tell the Reason, lest Captain Swan should come to hear of it.

So we left Captain Swan and about 36 Men ashore in the City, and 6 or 8 that run away; and about 16 we had buried there, the most of which died by Poison. The Natives are very expert at Poisoning, and do it upon small occasions: Nor did our Men want for giving Offence, through their general Rogueries, and sometimes by dallying too familiar with their Women, even before their Faces. Some of their Poisons are slow and lingering; for we had some now aboard who were Poison'd there; but died not till some Months after.[43]

Mr. Coppinger travelled widely about the East Indies: We hear of him in Manila,

whence he throws us the prettiest bit of news about another impromptu confrére:

Mr. Coppinger, our Surgeon, . . . made a voyage hither (to Manila) from Porto Nova, a Town on the Coast of Coromandel, in a Portuguese Ship, as I think. Here he found 10 or 12 of Captain Swan's Men; some of those that we left at Mindanao. For after he came from thence, they brought a Proe there, by the Instigation of an Irish Man, who went by the name of John Fitz-Gerald, a person that spoke Spanish very well; and so in this their Proe they came hither. They had been here but 18 months when Mr. Coppinger arrived here, and Mr. Fitz-Gerald had in this time gotten a Spanish Mustesa Woman to Wife, and a good Dowry with her. He then professed Physick and Surgery, and was highly esteemed among the Spaniards for his supposed knowledge in those Arts; for being always troubled with sore Shins while he was with us, he kept some Plaisters and Salves by him; and with these he set up upon his bare natural stock of knowledge, and his experience in Kibes. But then he had a very great stock of Confidence withal, to help out the other; and being an Irish Roman Catholick, and having the Spanish language, he had a great advantage of all his Consorts; and he alone lived well there of them all.[44]

A jolly, cunning rogue, Mr. Fitz-Gerald, with his Kibes, his Spanish Mustesa, his Dowry and his Salves and Plaisters, setting out his shingle in Manila 250 years in advance of his natural successors.

Mr. Coppinger and Dampier were much alike in their scientific tastes and their gravity. The companionship of the mutineers grew more and more irksome; their only thoughts were to get away; they were better scientists than pirates. In May of 1687 they were at Pulo Condore, an island off the coast of Cambodia.

While we stayed here Herman Coppinger our Surgeon went ashore, intending to live here; but Captain Read sent some Men to fetch him again. I had the same Thoughts, and would have gone ashore too, but waited for a more convenient place. For neither he nor I, when we were last on board at Mindanao, had any

---

[43] Dampier, I, 376.

[44] Dampier, I, 386–387.

knowledge of the Plot that was laid to leave Captain Swan, and run away with the Ship; and being sufficiently weary of this mad Crew we were willing to give them the slip at any place from whence we might hope to get a passage to an English Factory.[45]

They tried to get away again at the Nicobar Islands. When the ship was ready to sail Dampier got up his chest and bedding and desired the Captain to leave him ashore. He did leave him, but soon sent four or five armed men after him to fetch him aboard again. When he came aboard:

Found the Ship in an uproar. For there were 3 Men more, who taking Courage by my example, desired leave also to accompany me. One of them was the Surgeon, Mr. Coppinger. . . . But Capt. Read and his Crew would not part with the Surgeon. At last the Surgeon leapt into the Canoe, and taking up my Gun, swore he would go ashore, and that if any Man did oppose it, he would shoot him. But John Oliver, who was then Quarter Master, leapt into the Canoe, taking hold of him, took away the Gun, and with the help of two or three more, they dragged him again into the Ship.

They finally let Dampier and two others go, who later made their way to Sumatra, but the Surgeon they forced to stay.

Now we were Men enough to defend our selves against the Natives of this Island, if they should prove our Enemies: though if none of these Men had come ashore to me, I should not have feared any danger. Nay, perhaps less, because I should have been cautious of giving any offence to the Natives: and I am of the Opinion, that there are no People in the World so barbarous as to kill a single Person that falls accidentally into their Hands, or comes to live among them; except they have before been injured, by some outrage, or violence committed against them. Yet even then, or afterwards, if a Man could but preserve his Life from their first rage, and come to treat with them (which is the hardest thing, because their way is usually to abscond, and rushing suddenly upon their Enemy to kill him at unawares) one

might, by some slight, insinuate ones self into their Favours again.[46]

Mr. Coppinger did get away at last. The mutineers intended to sail to Persia, but being unable to weather Ceylon they sought refuge on the coast of Coromandel. Coppinger and another man left "this mad fickle crew" and went to the Danes at Trangambar (Tranquebar) who received them kindly. Here they lived very well. Coppinger engaged as surgeon on a Danish vessel, and sailed to Jihore on the Malacca coast to load pepper.

This is the last we hear of him. A quiet, serious-minded man, glad to get quit of the "mad fickle crew" with whom he had embarked.

There is not room to follow the fortunes of more of these rover surgeons, but we must consider some of the true pirates. They were a different breed; cut-throat, murdering rascals and knaves.

The exploits of the older English sea-rovers and buccaneers fire one with admiration; their ferocity and knaveries one condones. They were bred in a school of terror. It is difficult for us, nurslings of a soft age, to put ourselves in the old sailor-man's place; to picture the life and turn of mind and thought of these unlettered fighters, starving or subsisting for weeks together on rotten meat and rum, flogged with a rope's end at a tyrant captain's whim, sore and bloated with scurvy and syphilis, scabrous with lice and the itch. The natural recourse of such men's minds was drink, for that made merry men of poor tortured beasts. To see others suffer cannot have affected them much, for what did they not continually suffer themselves; to see others die (how often had not they seen their own shipmates die?) of wanton cruelty, starvation, hardships and disease. If they were fierce, their foe was fiercer; and if Henry Morgan put up the friars and nuns of Puerto Bello as a fence to his own pirates for the Spaniards to shoot at when he stormed the forts, the Grand Inquisitor

45 Dampier, I, 399.

46 Dampier, I, 470–471.

of Seville dealt no more gently, although perhaps more pompously and formally, with such English seamen as fell into his hands. If the old sea-rovers and buccaneers were cruel and terrible to their foes, cruel and terrible were the hardships they themselves endured. Their war was legitimate war, and their foes legitimate foes (in their eyes at least); they endured and inflicted cruelties and terrors in pursuit of them.

Not so with the pirates. With the exception of Captain Bartholomew Roberts (and Lafitte who was as much of a privateer and patriot as a pirate) there was scarcely a one who at the generous moment did not show himself a coward; their cruelties were those of maniacs and devils, hellish wantonnesses that one cannot find a place for among Englishmen. Theirs was the savagery of wolves, when the overpowering odds were on their side, or when they were brought to bay. From equal combat with men of their own race they turned tail and fled. Their cruelties were those of the Orient, or of the ancient Slavs and Vandals: tearing men's hearts out and roasting them alive, dragging out their testicles with a rope, cutting their ears and lips off and slashing open their bellies. One turns from them with abhorrence.

These sea-devils too had their doctors.

Among the worst of them was one Captain Ned Low. Low was bred a Westminster pickpocket, petty rogue and thief. He came to Boston and was married there in 1714. Soon after, his wife bore him a daughter and died in childbirth. Amid all his maniacal cruelties Low would never force a married man, and mention of his daughter would bring tears to his eyes. In 1722 he began his career of piracy and for two years terrorized the Atlantic from Newfoundland to the West Indies and eastward to the Azores. August, 1722, found him at the Azores, where he took seven vessels, among them a French ship. He transferred the crew to a launch, all except the cook, whom he declared to be a "greasy fellow who would fry well." He tied him to the main-

mast and set fire to the ship. Soon after a Captain Carter in the "Wright" galley sailed by. Carter resisted capture, so Low cut and mangled the passengers most cruelly; two Catholic friars he triced up to the end of the mainyard until they were near dead, when he let them down, repeating this sport again and again. One of the pirates saw a Portuguese passenger looking on in terror: he disemboweled him with a cutlass because he "didn't like his looks." Low himself was struck on the chin by a blow intended for another passenger. The blow laid open his teeth. His surgeon was called to stitch it up, but Low found fault with the way the job was done. The surgeon therefore hit him on the jaw with his fist and tore the stitches out again: "Go to Hell and sew up your own chops," said the doctor.

Sailing back to Brazil, Low fell in with a Portuguese vessel whose unfortunate captain slung his treasure of 11,000 moidores out of the cabin window in a sack. When he saw that capture was inevitable, he cut the rope and dropped the treasure into the sea. Low heard of it: he tied the wretched man to the mast, slashed off his lips with a cutlass, broiled them, peppered them and made the mate of the captured vessel eat them hot.

He sailed from Brazil to some of the smaller isles off the Venezuelan coast where, through drunkenness or ignorance, he turned his vessel turtle while trying to careen her. He and his surgeon were in the cabin when the sea gushed in; they both bolted out of one of the ports together. Low got out but the doctor was carried under by the force of the waters "upon which Low nimbly run his Arm into the Port and caught hold of his Shoulder and drew him out, and so saved him," the account says. His vessel was lost.

Cruising about the French West Indies it came into his head that he wanted a doctor's chest, so he put four French captives aboard a prize sloop and sent them off to St. Thomas to tell the Governor that if he'd not sell him a good chest for the money his captives brought with them he'd kill all the Frenchmen and burn ten or more French vessels that he then had in his hands. His captives returned with the chest.

We have no clear account of Low's end. It is probable that his crew cast him adrift for murdering his quartermaster in his sleep and that he was taken and hanged by the French on the Isle of Martinique.

With Low there sailed Charles Harris. Harris was second mate of a captured vessel; he joined the pirates and Low gave him command of a prize, the sloop Ranger. On June 10, 1723, they were sighted between Cape Delaware and Block Island by the man-of-war Greyhound, Peter Solgard commander, of the New York station which had received advice of their being off the coast. Captain Solgard stood to the South and led them on by pretending to run away. Suddenly he turned and opened fire. The two pirates were more than a match for him, but Low fled while Captain Solgard engaged Harris in the Ranger. He took the Ranger and her crew and brought them into Boston, thirty-seven in all, where they were tried and hanged. Dow and Edmunds give an account of the trial. In the list of prisoners there is mentioned "John Hinchard, Doctor, age 22, Place of Birth, Near Edinburgh, N. Brit." This name, however, does not appear among the reports of the trials; here the doctor's name is John Kencate. Dow and Edmunds' report reads:

The next morning John Kencate, the doctor on board the "Ranger" was brought to trial. The Advocate General stated that although the prisoner "used no arms, was not harness'd (as they term it) but was a forc'd man; yet if he received part of their plunder, was not under a constant durance, did at any time approve, or join'd in their villanies, his guilt is at least equal to the rest; the Doctor being ador'd among 'em as the pirates' God for in him they chiefly confide for their cure and life, and in this trust and dependence it is, that they enterprise these horrid depredations not to be heightened by aggravation, or lessened by any excuse."

Capt. John Welland deposed, and that he saw the Doctor aboard the Ranger; he seem'd not to rejoice when he was taken but solitary, and he was inform'd on board he was a forc'd man; and that he never signed the articles as he heard of, and was now on board the deponants ship.

John Ackin Mate and John Mudd Carpenter, swore they saw the prisoner at the Bar walking forwards and backwards disconsolately on board the Ranger.

Archibald Fisher Physician and Chirurgion on board the said Greyhound Man-of-War deposed, that when the prisoner at the Bar was taken and brought aboard the King's ship he searched his medicaments, and the instruments, and found but very few medicaments, and the instruments very mean and bad.

Others testified that the doctor was forced on board, by Low, and that he never signed articles so far as they knew or heard, but used to spend much of his time in reading, and was very courteous to the prisoners taken by Low and his company, and that he never shared with him.

The Doctor himself said that he was chirurgion of the *Sycamore*—Galley, Andrew Scot, master, and was taken out of that ship in September last at Bonavista, one of the Cape de Verde Islands, by Low and Company, who detained him ever since, and that he never shared with them, nor signed their articles.

The court then cleared the doctor . . . [47]

Of Peter Scudamore, Captain Bartholomew Roberts' surgeon, we have some detail. Roberts sailed from London in 1719 in an honest employ, as second mate of the ship Princess. His ship was taken by the pirate Howel Davis off the coast of Guinea the February following. Six weeks later, Howel Davis having been killed, Roberts was elected commander. He was a stern and bloody man, the prototype of the picture-book pirate. Coming into an engagement he was wont to array himself in a rich crimson damask waistcoat and breeches, and to hang a gold chain with a diamond cross about his neck. Two pairs of pistols hung at the end of a silken sling flung over his shoulders. Stern and bloody, as befitted his calling, he seems not to have committed the wanton atrocities of other pirate captains.

[47] Dow and Edmunds. Pirates of the New England Coast. Salem, Mass., 1923, p. 302–303.

The year 1720 he spent in cruising about Brazil and Newfoundland and the West Indies. He narrowly escaped capture at the Barbadoes and the Isle of Martinique so that all Barbadoes and Martinican men were hated by him ever after. He had a flag made showing his figure, a flaming sword in hand, standing with a skull under each foot; the skulls were labelled A. B. H. and A. M. H., signifying A Barbadian's and A Martinican's Head. This flag he called the "Jolly Roger." In 1721 he sailed up and down the Guinea coast robbing and plundering and laying waste. The British man-of-war Swallow gave him chase and engaged him off Cape Lopez. They first drew on a smaller one of Roberts' ships, called the Ranger, and took her with her crew of sixteen Frenchmen, twenty Negroes, and seventy-seven English. While the Swallow was sending her boat to fetch off the prisoners, a great blast of smoke was seen pouring out of the Ranger's cabin. Half a dozen of the most desperate of the pirates, all hope of escape being gone, had fired their pistols into what was left of their powder. It was not enough to blow up the ship, but maimed and burnt them horribly. The Swallow's surgeon, seeing a pirate named Roger Ball distressingly burnt and sitting sullenly in a corner, asked him how he came to be so burnt and offered to dress his wounds for him. Ball swore that he should not and that if anything were applied to him he would tear it off. Nevertheless the surgeon dressed him, although with much trouble. At night Ball fell into a kind of delirium, probably a delirium tremens, and raved on the bravery of Roberts; so he was lashed down upon the forecastle. Resisting restraint, he was tied all the more severely, and his flesh being sore and tender with the powder burns he died the next day "of a mortification."

Four days later the Swallow engaged Roberts' own ship, the Royal Fortune. The crew who sighted the Swallow warned Roberts, but he was at breakfast with the captain of a recent prize and would take no heed. He fought very desperately until a grape-shot struck him directly on the throat and killed him.

He settled himself on the tackles of a gun, which one Stephenson from the helm observing ran to his assistance and not perceiving him wounded, swore at him and bid him stand up and fight like a man; but when he found his mistake and that his captain was certainly dead, he gushed into tears and wished the next shot might be his lot. They presently threw him overboard, with his arms and ornaments on, according to the repeated requests he made in his lifetime.[48]

Roberts frankly owned that he had turned pirate to get rid of the disagreeable superiority of some of the masters he had been acquainted with and the love of novelty and change maritime peregrination had accustomed him to.

"In an honest service," said he, "there is thin commons, low wages, and hard labour; in this plenty and satiety, pleasure and ease, liberty and power; and who would not balance credits on this side when all the hazard that is run for it, at worst, is only a fore-look or two at choking." He is said never to have forced a man into piracy.

With Roberts' death the life and soul went out of his crew; they deserted their quarters and stood stupidly by; their mainmast was shot by the board and they surrendered and called for quarter.

On board the Royal Fortune were 157 men, whereof forty-five were negroes, and £2,000 in gold dust; only three men were killed in action.

Among the prisoners taken by the Swallow were three surgeons: Adam Comry, taken in the Ranger, joined from Ship Elizabeth, Capt. Sharp, January, 1722; Peter Scudamore, taken in the Royal Fortune, joined from Mercy galley at Calabar, October, 1721; and George Wilson, joined from Ship Tarlton of Liverpool, January, 1722.

The records of the trials stand as a monument to the fairness and despatch of English

[48] Buccaneers and Marooners of America. Ed. and illus. by Howard Pyle. London, 1897, p. 328.

justice. They were held at the Factory of the Royal African Company at Cape Corso Castle (Cape Coast Castle). They were begun March 28, 1722; the first six pirates were hanged five days later without the gates of the castle and within the flood marks of the tide. The account stands: Acquitted seventy-four; hanged, thirty-two; respited, two; commuted to servitude, twenty; to the Marshalsea, seventeen; killed in the Ranger, ten; in the Fortune, three; died in the passage to Cape Corso, thirteen; died afterwards in the Castle, four; negroes seventy. Total 276.

"The country wherein they happened to be tried," the narrative says, "is among other happinesses exempted from lawyers and law-books." A commission of five was therefore chosen, and any three commissioners were empowered to call to their assistance a number of qualified persons to make the court always consist of seven. The commissioners found some difficulty in finding a proper indictment. Their oath ran "that they have no interest, directly or indirectly, in the ship or goods, for the robbery of which the party stands accused." As servants of the Royal African Company, however, they had an interest in the cargoes captured by the pirates. Furthermore it was impossible, particularly to specify in the charge as they were enjoined to do, "the circumstances of time, place, etc." for the various piracies. The indictment, therefore, was made on offering resistance to the King's Ship Swallow, and not for acts of piracy committed upon merchantmen.

The court considered whether or not they should pardon one Jo. Dennis who had early offered himself as King's evidence. They concluded no; although they lost by it "those great helps he could have afforded . . . because it looked like compounding with a man to swear falsely."

And finally . . . "to approve their clemency, it looking arbitrary on the lives of men to lump them to the gallows in such a summary way as must have been done had they solely adhered to the Swallow's

charge, they resolved to come to particular trials."

That the prisoners might not be ignorant whereon to answer, and so have all fair advantages to excuse and defend themselves, the court farther agreed with justice and equanimity to hear any evidence that could be brought to weaken or corroborate the three circumstances that complete a pirate: first, being a volunteer amongst them at the beginning; secondly, being a volunteer at the taking or robbing of any ship; or, lastly, voluntarily accepting a share in the booty of those that did; for by a parity of reason where these actions were of their own disposing, and yet committed by them it must be believed their hearts and hands joined together in what they acted against his Majesty's ship the Swallow.[49]

There is justice and fairness; in that court of commissioners, themselves but lately escaped with their lives from the hands of the men they had up before them for trial; sitting on a far African Coast, without fear of surveillance or check from the Mother Country, free to act as they would. Just and fair because they were Englishmen and wanted to be just and fair, and not because anyone or anything made them be so.

Of one of the surgeon-prisoners, Adam Comry, we have not many particulars; pictures of the two others, Scudamore and Wilson, we can construct in sufficient detail. Adam Comry was surgeon to the ship Elizabeth, Jo. Sharp master, taken by Roberts off the African coast in January, 1722. He was forced into the pirate service by Scudamore and served on board the Ranger. At the trial of the pirates he was acquitted. He seems to have been a kind and decent man, and to have been heartily uncomfortable in the company he was in. And well he might, with the ghost of a noose tickling at his neck.

George Wilson and Peter Scudamore were thorough rogues.

[49] Trial. Quoted by Pyle, Buccaneers and Marooners of America, p. 335–336.

Wilson sailed as surgeon to the Ship Tarlton of Liverpool, Capt. John Tarlton master, which Roberts fell in with and captured near Cape Lahou off the Ivory Coast of Africa early in January, 1722. At this trial he testified that after he had been aboard the pirate vessel for a day or two, Captain Roberts told him "to his sorrow" that he was to stay there and ordered him to fetch his chest from the Tarlton:

Which opportunity he took to make his escape; for the boat's crew happening to consist of five French and one Englishman, all as willing as himself, they agreed to push the boat on shore and trust themselves with the negroes of Cape Montzerado. Hazardous, not only in respect of the dangerous seas that run there, but the inhumanity of the natives, who sometimes take a liking to human carcasses. Here he remained five months, till Thomas Tarlton, brother to his captain, chanced to put into the road for trade, to whom he represented his hardships and starving condition; but was in an unchristian manner, both refused a release of this captivity, or so much as a small supply of biscuit and salt meat, because, as he said, he had been among the pirates. A little time after this the master of a French ship paid a ransom for him and took him off; but, by reason of a nasty leprous indisposition he had contracted by hard and bad living, was, to his great misfortune, set ashore at Sestos again.[50]

Other witnesses deposed (and judging by the joy he showed at being captured by the Pirates a second time their version seems the more likely), that the doctor did not "seize the opportunity to escape," but that his boat was swept ashore by a strong wind and that he was held there by the natives; and that it was this accident and not his intention that kept him from getting aboard the pirates again.

Captain Sharp of the Elizabeth met him at Sestos and "generously procured his release" buying him from his negro captors for a ransom of goods to the value of three pounds five shillings. Sharp took Wilson's note for the money; but the note did not

much matter. As they left the ship after the capture by the pirates, Wilson asked the Captain whether the pirates had the note or no. And Sharp not being able to say, he replied, "It's no matter, Mr. Sharp, I believe I shall hardly ever come to England to pay it," which prophecy fell true, as we shall see later.

Captain Sharp testified at the trial that he thought he had done a charitable act in ransoming the Doctor till "meeting with one Captain Canning he was asked why he would release such a rogue as Wilson was? for that he had been a volunteer with the pirates out of John Tarlton."

Captain Sharp's ship Elizabeth was captured by Roberts a little later, so that Wilson fell into the pirates' hands a second time. Sharp and his surgeon Adam Comry must have rued the day they ransomed this doctor from the negroes. Three pounds five was much too good a price to have paid. Neither his legitimate master nor the pirates seem to have had a good word for him.

At the trial his colleague Comry testified:

Although the prisoner had, on account of his indisposition and want, received many civilities from him before meeting with the pirates, he yet understood it was through his and Scudamore's means that he had been compelled among them. The prisoner was very alert and cheerful, he says, at meeting with Roberts, hailed him, told him he was glad to see him, and would come on board presently, borrowing of the deponent a clean shirt and drawers, for his better appearance and reception; he signed their Articles willingly, and used arguments with him to do the same, saying, they should make their voyage in eight months to Brazil, share six or seven hundred pounds a man, and then break up. Again, when the crew came to an election of a chief surgeon, and this deponent was set up with the others, Wilson told him, he hoped he would carry it from Scudamore, for that a quarter share (which they had more than others) would be worth looking after; but the deponent missed the preferment, by the good will of the Ranger's people, who, in general, voted for Scudamore, to get rid of him, the chief surgeon being always to remain with the commodore.

[50] Pyle, p. 370-371.

It appeared likewise by the evidence of Captain Jo. Trahern, Tho. Castel, and others, who had been taken by the pirates, and thence had opportunities of observing the prisoner's conduct, that he seemed thoroughly satisfied with that way of life, and was particularly intimate with Roberts; they often scoffing at the mention of a man-of-war, and saying, if they should meet with any of the turnip-man's ships, they would blow up and go to h—l all together. Yet setting aside these silly freaks to recommend himself, his laziness had got him many enemies; even Roberts told him, on the complaint of a wounded man, whom he had refused to dress, that he was a double rogue to be there a second time, and threatened to cut his ears off.

The evidence further assured the court, from Captain Thomas Tarlton, that the prisoner was taken out of his brother's ship, some months before, a first time, and being forward to oblige his new company, had presently asked for the pirates' boat to fetch his medicine-chest away, when the wind and current proving too hard to contend with, he was drove on shore at Cape Montzerado.[51]

When he got aboard Roberts' ship the second time he found Thomas Tarlton, brother of his old captain John Tarlton, a fellow prisoner. He had met Thomas Tarlton at Cape Montzerado when he was cast ashore there among the natives and Tarlton had refused to ransom him. Here then was a chance for evening an old score. The doctor instigated the pirates against Tarlton, who was immediately, "in a most sad manner misused and beat, and had been shot, through the fury and rage of some of those fellows, if the town-side (i.e., Liverpool) men had not hid him in a staysail under the bowsprit, for Moody and Harper with their pistols cocked searched every corner of the ship to find him, and came to the deponent's hammock, whom they had like fatally to have mistaken for Tarlton, but on his calling out they found their error, and left him with this comfortable anodyne, that 'he was the honest fellow who brought the doctor.'"[52]

The doctor put up a lame and shifty defence at his trial. He said:

[51] Pyle. *Op. cit.*, p. 368–369.
[52] Pyle. *Op. cit.*, p. 367–368.

Ill-luck threw him a second time into the pirates' hands, in this ship Elizabeth, where he met Thomas Tarlton, and thoughtlessly used some reproaches of him for his severe treatment at Montzerado; but protests without design his words should have had so bad a consequence; for Roberts took upon him, as a dispenser of justice, the correction of Mr. Tarlton, beating him unmercifully; and, he hopes it will be believed, contrary to any intention of his it should so happen, because, as a stranger, he might be supposed to have no influence, and believes there were some other motives for it. He can not remember he expressed himself glad to see Roberts this second time, or that he dropped those expressions about Comry, as are sworn; but if immaturity of judgment had occasioned him to slip rash and inadvertent words, or that he had paid any undue compliments to Roberts, it was to ingratiate himself, as every prisoner did, for a more civil treatment, and in particular to procure his discharge, which he had been promised, and was afraid would have been revoked, if such a person as Comry did not remain there to supply his room; and of this, he said, all the gentlemen (meaning the pirates) could witness for him.

He urged also his youth in excuse for his rashness. The first time he had been with them (only a month in all), and that in no military employ; but in particular the service he had done in discovering the design the pirates had to rise in their passage on board the Swallow.[53]

And so the doctor was judged guilty.

His execution, however, was respited "till the King's pleasure be known," because the commander of the Swallow declared that Wilson had given him the first notice of a plot of the pirate prisoners to rise and seize the vessel while being conveyed from Wydah Road to Cape Coast Castle.

His sentence was never executed; he died abroad, and did never come again to England to pay his note to Captain Sharp.

A memory of roguery and laziness and knavery, you leave behind you, young Doctor Wilson. Your colleague Comry in the kindness of his heart fits you out with a clean shirt and drawers so that you may appear presentably before your pirate captain, you return his kindness by having him forced aboard against his will. You

[53] Pyle. *Op. cit.*, p. 371–372.

refuse to dress the wounded, and even your new pirate master tells you that you are a double rogue to be with him a second time and threatens to cut your ears off. All that saves your neck from the rope is betrayal of your fellow prisoners' plans for freedom.

Better for your reputation you had stayed among the negroes at Cape Montzerado and rotted there of your "nasty leprous indisposition."

The third of the doctor trio is Peter Scudamore, a blustering bragadoccio rascal, full of windy schemes, a Welshman; his last moments find him taking solace in religion; he sticks his neck into the hangman's noose chanting the thirty-first Psalm. Here is the testimony at his trial:

PETER SCUDAMORE

Harry Glasby, Jo. Wingfield, and Nicholas Brattle, depose thus much as to his being a volunteer with the pirates from Captain Rolls at Calabar. First, that he quarreled with Moody (one of the heads of the gang), and fought with him because he opposed his going, asking Rolls in a leering manner whether he would not be so kind as to put him into the Gazette when he came home. And, at another time, when he was going from the pirate ship in his boat a tornado arose. "I wish," says he, "the rascal may be drowned, for he is a great rogue, and has endeavoured to do me all the ill offices he could among these gentlemen" (i.e., pirates).

And secondly, that he had signed the pirates' Articles with a great deal of alacrity, and gloried in having been the first surgeon that had done so (for before this it was their custom to change their surgeons when they desired it, after having served a time, and never obliged them to sign, but he was resolved to break through this for the good of those who were to follow), swearing immediately upon it, he was now, he hoped, as great a rogue as any of them.

Captain Jo. Trahern and George Fenn, his mate, deposed the prisoner to have taken out of the King Solomon their surgeon's capital instruments, some medicines and a backgammon table, which latter became the means of a quarrel between one Wincon and he, whose property they should be, and were yielded to the prisoner.

Jo. Sharp, master of the Elizabeth, heard the prisoner ask Roberts' leave to force Comry, his surgeon, from him, which was accordingly done, and with him carried also some of the ship's medicines; but what gave a fuller proof of the dishonesty of his principles was the treacherous design he had formed of running away with the prize in her passage to Cape Corso, though he had been treated with all humanity and very unlike a prisoner on account of his employ and better education, which had rendered him less to be suspected.

Mr. Child (acquitted) deposed that in their passage from the Island of St. Thomas in the Fortune prize, this prisoner was several times tempting him into measures of rising with the negroes, and killing the Swallow's people, showing him how easily the white men might be demolished, and a new company raised at Angola, and that part of the coast. "For," says he, "I understand how to navigate a ship, and can soon teach you to steer; and is it not better to do this than to go back to Cape Corso and be hanged and sun-dried?" To which the deponent replying he was not afraid of being hanged, Scudamore bid him be still, and no harm could come to him; but before the next day evening, which was the designed time of executing this project, this deponent discovered it to the officer, and assured him Scudamore had been talking all the preceding night to his negroes in Angolan language.

Isaac Burnet heard the prisoner ask James Harris, a pirate (left with the wounded in the prize), whether he was willing to come into the project of running away with the ship, and endeavour the raising of a new company, but turned the discourse to horse racing as the deponent crept nigher; he acquainted the officer with what he had heard, who kept the people under arms all night, their apprehensions of the negroes being groundless; for many of them having lived a long time in this piratical way, were, by the thin commons they were now reduced to, as ripe for mischief as any.

The prisoner in his defence said he was a forced man from Captain Rolls in October last, and if he had not shown such a concern as became him at the alteration he must remark the occasion to be the disagreement and enmity between them; but that both Roberts and Val. Ashplant threatened him into signing their Articles, and that he did it in terror.

The King Solomon and Elizabeth medicine-chests he owns he plundered by order of Hunter, the then chief surgeon, who, by the pirates' laws, always directs in this province, and Mr. Child (though acquitted) had, by the same orders, taken out a whole French medicine-chest, which he must be sensible for me as well as for himself we neither of us dared to have denied; it was their being the proper judges made so ungrateful an office imposed. If after this he was elected chief surgeon himself both Comry and Wilson were set up also and it might have been their chance to have carried it, and as much out of their power to have refused.

As to the attempt of rising and running away with the prize, he denies it altogether as untrue; a few foolish words, but only by way of supposition, that if the negroes should take it in their heads (considering the weakness and ill look-out that was kept), it would have been an easy matter in his opinion for them to have done it; but that he encouraged such a thing was false; his talking to them in the Angolan language was only a way of spending his time, and trying his skill to tell twenty, he being incapable of further talk. As to his understanding navigation, he had frequently acknowledged it to the deponent Child, and wonders he should now so circumstantiate this skill against him. Guilty.[54]

He seems for all his alacrity in signing their Articles, to have been in no great favour with the pirates themselves. When it came to elect a chief surgeon, the choice lying between Scudamore and Comry, the crew of the Ranger voted for Scudamore. By this means they hoped to get him off their vessel and onto the Royal Fortune, the flagship of the pirate fleet; the rule being that the chief surgeon was always to stay with the commodore. Diplomats and politicians, those pirates.

The "old standers" among the pirates walked to the gallows without "as much concern as a man would express at travelling a bad road; nay, Simpson at seeing among the crowd a woman that he knew, said, "He had lain with that bitch three times and now she was come to see him hanged."

But others behaved with seeming devotion and penitence, among them Doctor Peter.

[54] Pyle. *Op. cit.*, p. 363–366.

Scudamore too lately discerned the folly and wickedness of the enterprise, that had chiefly brought him under sentence of death, from which, seeing there was no hopes of escaping, he petitioned for two or three days' reprieve, which was granted; and for that time applied himself incessantly to prayer and reading the Scriptures. He seemed to have a deep sense of his sins, of this in particular, and desired, at the gallows, they would have patience with him, to sing the first part of the thirty-first Psalm; which he did by himself throughout.[55]

In thee, O *Lord*, do I put my trust; let me never be ashamed; deliver me in thy righteousness.

Bow down thine ear to me; deliver me speedily; be thou my strong rock, for an house of defence to save me.

For thou art my rock and my fortress; therefore for thy name's sake lead me, and guide me.

Pull me out of the net that they have laid privily for me; for thou art my strength.

Into thine hand I commit my spirit; thou hast redeemed me, O *Lord*, God of truth.

I have hated them that trust lying vanities; but I trust in the LORD.

Thus sings the Doctor, the black cap over his head, his neck in the noose.

A trying time for the poor Welshman. Good-bye, Dr. Scudamore.

These few samples will do to sketch the sort of men who doctored the pirates and buccaneers. As men not so different from their present-day colleagues, all kinds: the grave, the blustering, the whimsical, the tranquil; the pompous, the cantankerous; the cock-sure, the lazy; the helpful, the kind; the roistering, the honest, and the knavish—all kinds but the picayune and the squeamish. Their surroundings may have fostered crime and sin, but no petty foibles; no paper rules and blanks to fill out, nor quarantines and surveys and public health regulations; only terrible foes, visible and invisible; terrible men, terrible disease, terrible tempests, heat, cold, hunger and thirst; terrible passion, greed, murder and savagery.

[55] Pyle. *Op cit.*, p. 382.

Coachwhip Publications

CoachwhipBooks.com

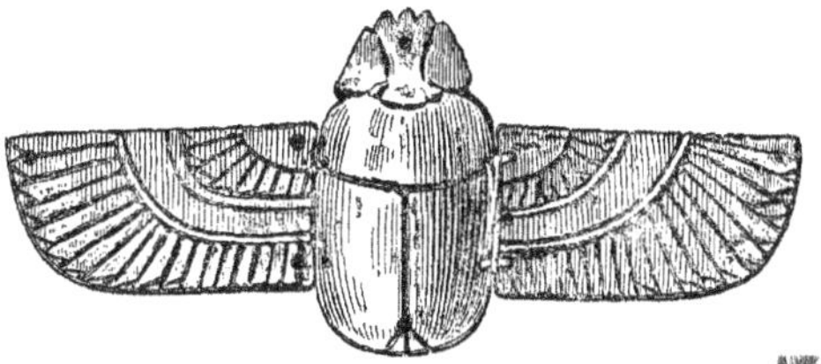

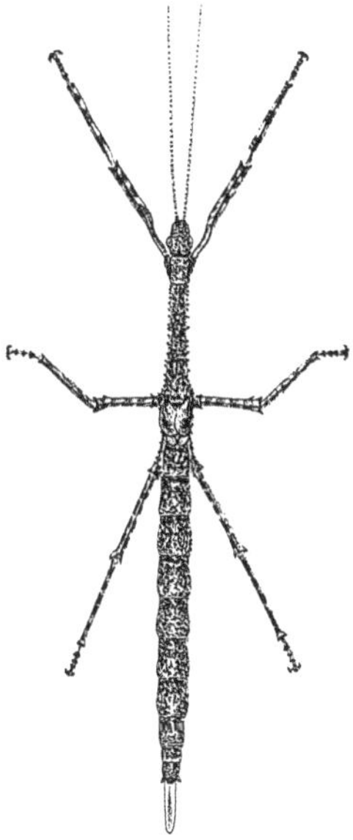

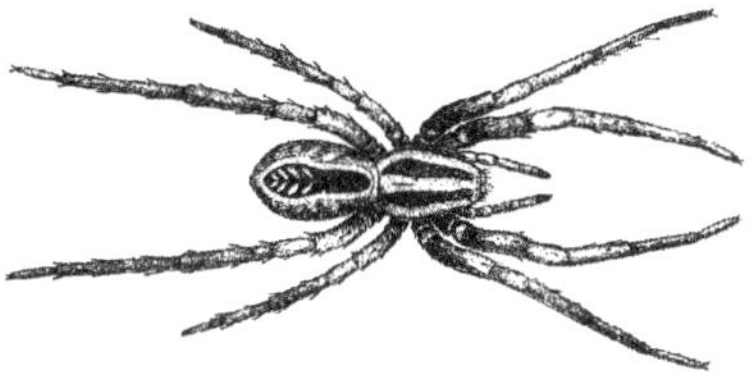

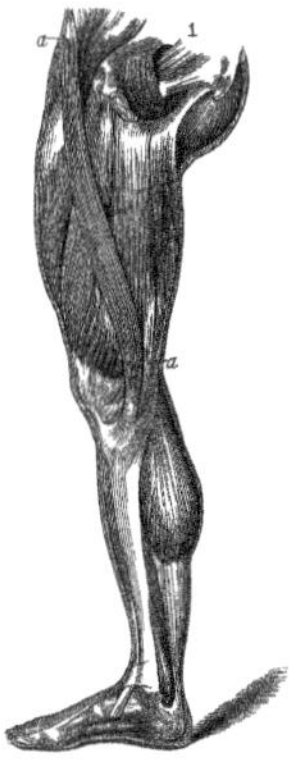

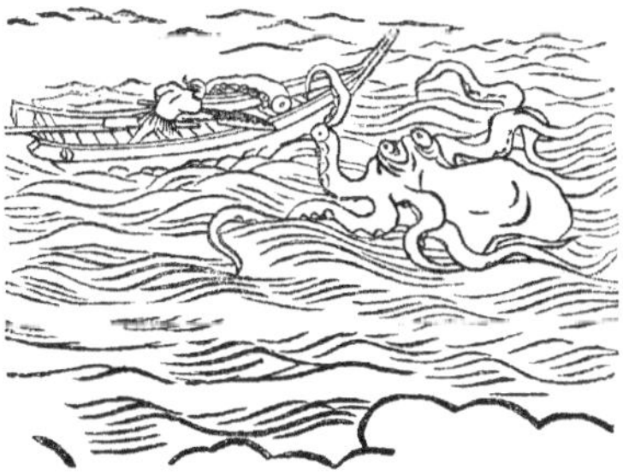

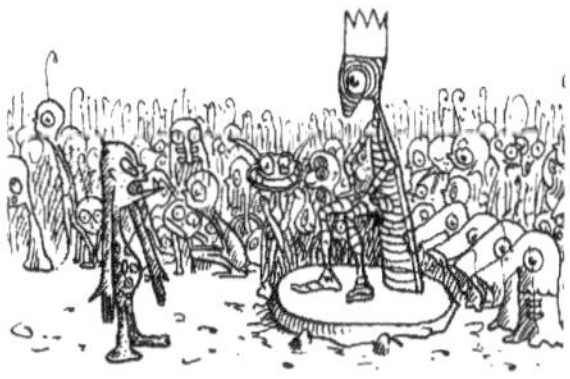

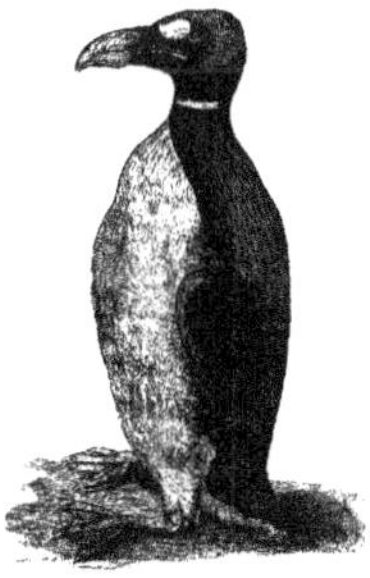

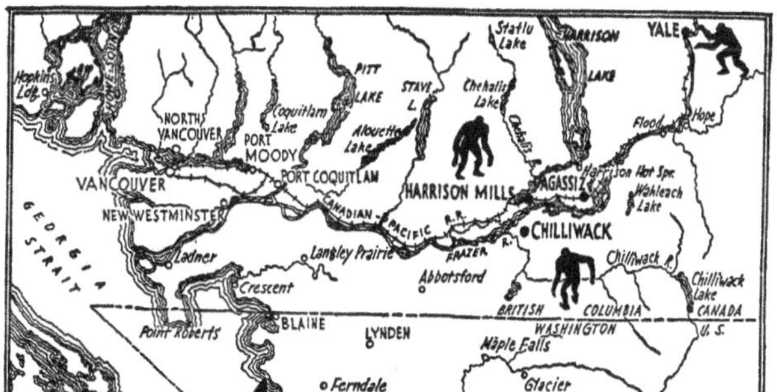

www.ingramcontent.com/pod-product-compliance
Lightning Source LLC
Chambersburg PA
CBHW081228040426
42445CB00016B/1919